COOKING FOR FERTILITY

Foods to Nourish Your Fertile Soul

by Kathryn Simmons Flynn

Foreword by Randine Lewis, Ph.D, L.Ac.

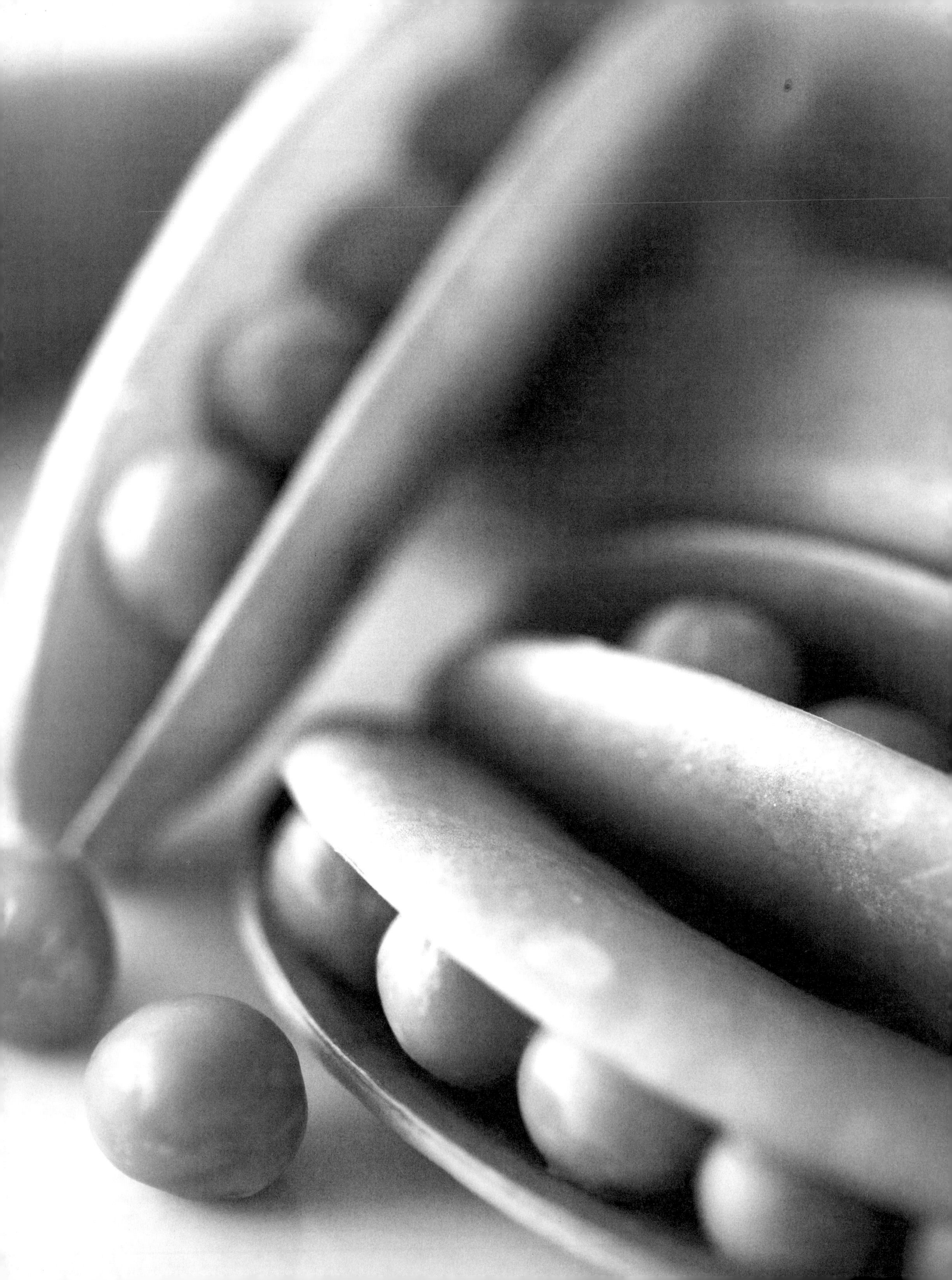

Praise for Fertility

Kathryn's ability to identify simple and wholesome foods that nourish the soul during the fertility journey is a direct reflection of her compassionate nature as a true healer. In my many years of clinical experience in not only the treatment of infertility but across my entire patient population, Kathryn's wisdom has always provided comfort, insight and results to patients who are in need of refuge. To think that they could find solace in the preparation of the food they eat and find themselves along the way is the greatest gift any healer can provide. This book is more then a collection of recipes, it is an offering to return to ourselves through our food and in the process become whole.

Dr. David A. Lundgren (RI)

Executive Director
The Fertile Soul's
Clinical Excellence in Fertility Professionals

In traditional Chinese Medicine (and in most indigenous cultures for that matter) food is considered sacred medicine. It is what the people use first to create subtle and profound changes in their body/mind. This deeply wise way of being in relationship with food is just beginning to be "discovered" here in the West.

And this is where Kathryn's book comes in: It provides the language and framework for you to begin to understand food and your Being from a holistic perspective. It is from this perspective that one enters into a truly wholesome and healing relationship with life itself.

As a holistic health care provider specializing in Chinese Medicine, I see first hand how important food preparations, interactions and choices are in creating vitality. If my patients desire to conceive, Cooking for Fertility is the first book that I recommend.

~Tiffany Pollard

Creator of Eating For Evolution and Synergy Wellness Center

What a treasure! This exquisite book is the long awaited answer to the search of so many women struggling with infertility! Kathryn has created these nurturing and healing recipes that offer comfort and entice the palette of women craving the essential sustenance that feeds mind, body and soul. These delicious dishes are served with gentle direction, generous options, and beautiful presentation. What an incredible resource for all those in the world of wellness supporting women on their journey to not only conceive and have healthy babies, but also to be healthy moms!

Michelle Galatoire

Life Coach, awomanswellness.com

Kathryn Simmons Flynn is conscious of the health and wellness connection between WHAT we eat and HOW we eat. Her holistic understanding of how our food and our eating behavior are tied to emotions is rooted in age-old healing traditions and modern science. Consciousness and resulting emotions, from tranquility to stress, affect the overall optimum operating of all of our vital functioning including reproductive health, pregnancy and post-partum strength. Cooking for Fertility offers recipes and insights to nourish body, spirit and soul, honoring our inner healing wisdom.

Caspar Poyck, C.Ht.

Culinary Life Coach
Consciously Culinary™

Kathryn Simmons Flynn's book provides much-needed simple, practical guidelines and recipes for eating to enhance fertility. Her advice is uncomplicated and easy to apply in real life. But more than this, she approaches diet and nutrition from an Eastern perspective, where foods are used to support, strengthen and balance one's body, mind and spirit.

My students over the years have commented that the yoga they learned while trying to get pregnant has brought them lifelong benefits. In the same way, not only will the information in Kathryn's book help women conceive, it will continue to benefit them and their families with better health throughout their lives, long after the baby arrives.

Lynn Jensen, RYT, MBA

Founder/Director, Yoga for Fertility

Before naturally conceiving my first son I turned to acupuncture after reading Randine Lewis' book "The Infertility Cure." This was after a miscarriage, 3 failed IUIs and the recommendation of IVF due to my age (36) and unexplained infertility after nearly two years of trying to conceive.

When we started trying for baby #2 two years later I was 39 with a High FSH (17.7) and was told I'd likely need donor eggs. After a phone consultation with Kathryn Flynn, which led to a complete change in diet, I again turned to acupuncture and conceived without medical intervention within a few months.

Our second miracle baby boy was born in May 2009. I'm truly grateful to the Fertile Soul program, as I believe the nutritional evaluation and recommendations and the faith in the process provided by "The Infertility Cure" helped pave our path to our darling sons.

E.M., California

I'M PREGNANT, Kathryn!!! Confirmed at my RE's (Reproductive Endocrinologist) office – and boy were they ever surprised! At age 42, I was told by my RE that, after 2 1/2 years of trying to get pregnant with one full year devoted to lots of drugs, 2 unsuccessful IUIs, and 1 unsuccessful IVF attempt, adoption or donor eggs were my only options. "Unexplained infertility" was my diagnosis. I walked away with tremendous anger and loads of anxiety. Then I met you and started our nutrition sessions once a month along with acupuncture and herbs. 5 months later, the miracle happened...I was pregnant...naturally!!

And much of what I learned in all this came from the practical insights and guidance of your wonderful cookbook. I would highly recommend your cookbook to anyone on the fertility journey as a complete resource guide to restoring reproductive balance and a healthy mindset. Thank you again and again for the gift you were to me in my journey to find wholeness and peace; I found both of these and, in the process, was blessed by the miracle of new life. Now 18 weeks pregnant, my husband and I eagerly await the arrival of our unexpected bundle of joy.

Much love and gratitude,

P.M., Illinois

I just wanted to let you know that I have been doing really well eating better. My sugar cravings are gone and I am beginning to really think before I eat. I feel better. I have more energy, am less bloated and my skin looks really good. Plus I know I have been shedding some weight, so that is the extra bonus to all of these great changes I'm experiencing!

K.W., California

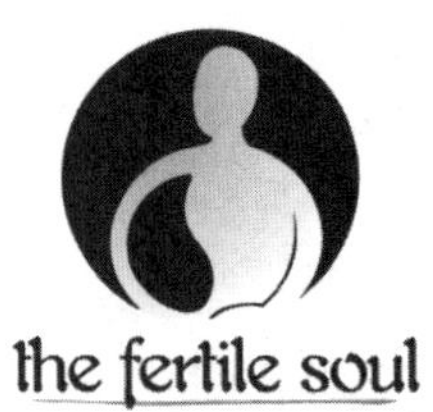

26 Glencove Drive
Arden, NC 28704

The information contained in this book is intended to be educational and not a diagnosis, prescription, or treatment of any health disorder whatsoever. This information should not replace consultation with a competent health care professional. The content of the book is intended to be used as an adjunct to a rational and responsible health care program prescribed by a professional health care practitioner. The author and publisher are no way liable for any misuse of the material.

Editor: Wendy Andersen
Copy editor & index: Doug Yonson
Cover & interior design: Gabriela Aparicio
Pictures: Kristen Bontadelli

For more information about bulk purchases please contact The Fertile Soul 1-866-469-3378
or coordinator@thefertilesoul.com

Published and Printed in the United States of America
Library of Congress Cataloguing-in-Publication Data: 2010920627
Flynn, Kathryn Simmons
Cooking for Fertility: Foods to Nourish Your Fertile Soul/Kathryn Simmons Flynn

1.2. I.
ISBN 978-0-615-33974-0+

"One cannot think well, love well, sleep well, if one has not dined well."

~Virgina Woolf

This book is dedicated to the amazing women in my family, including my grandmothers Margaret Hollingsworth and Margaret Jean Simmons, my aunt Margaret McElroy, my mother Lois Simmons and my sister Meghan, who all know that all food tastes good when made with love and laughter.

Contents

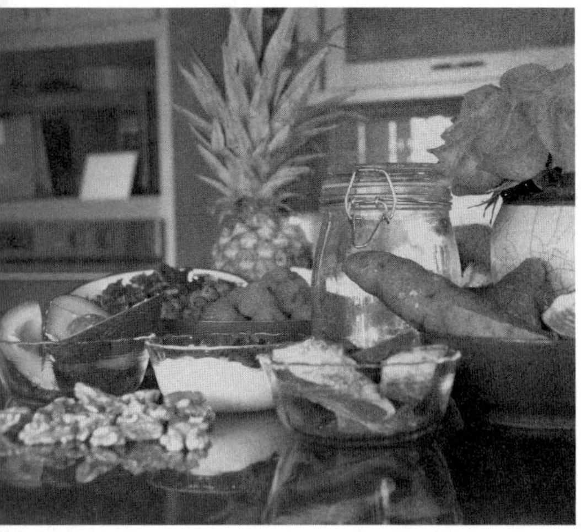

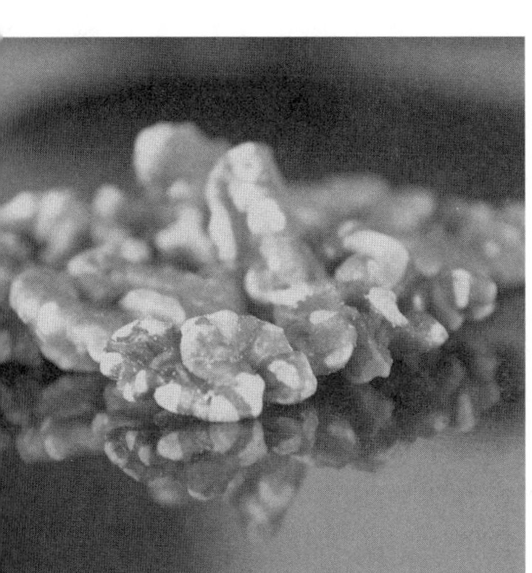

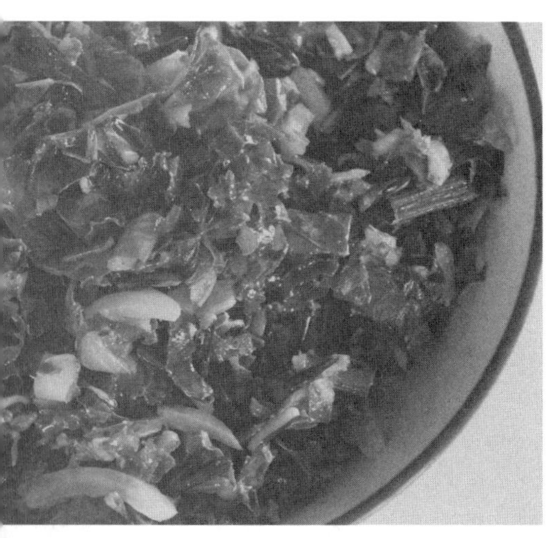

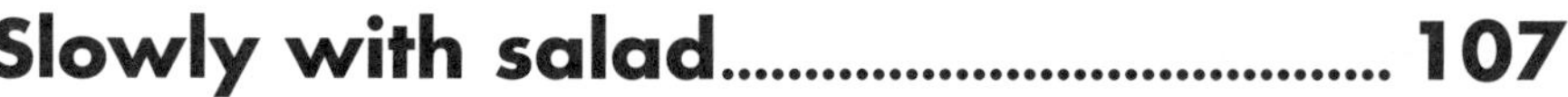

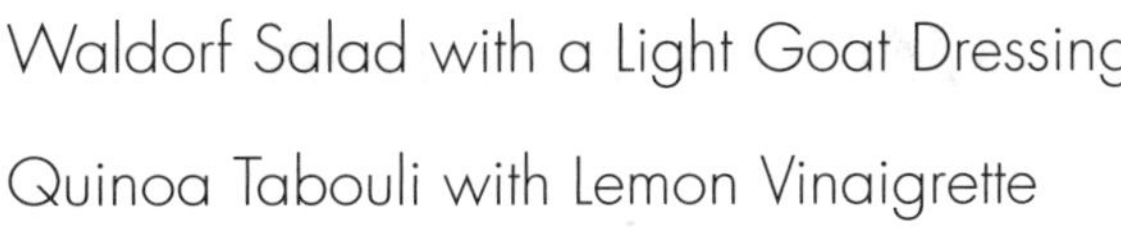

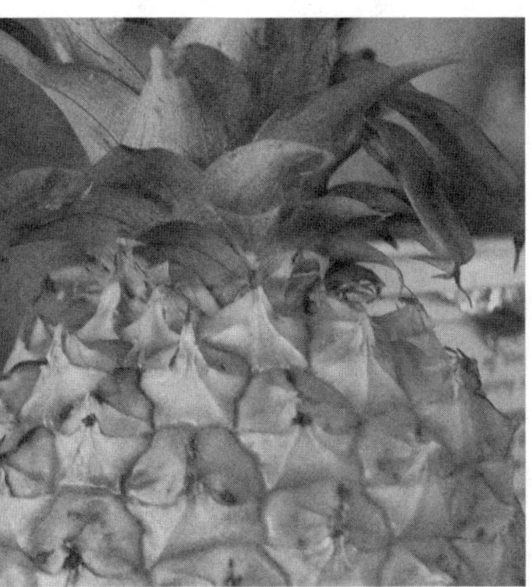

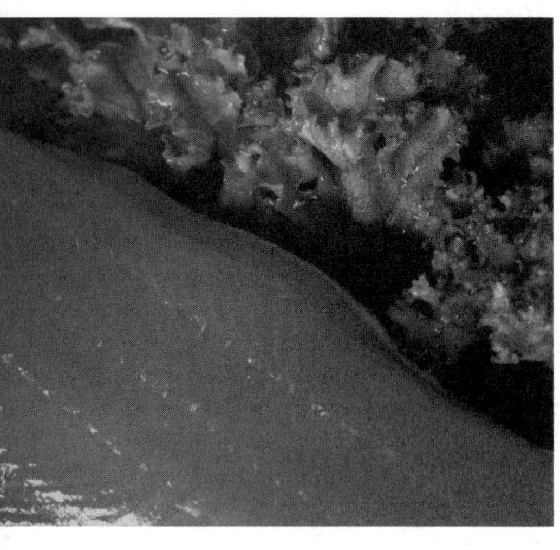

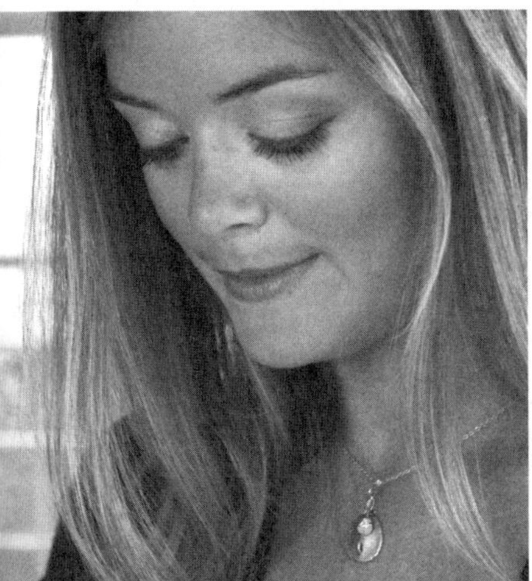

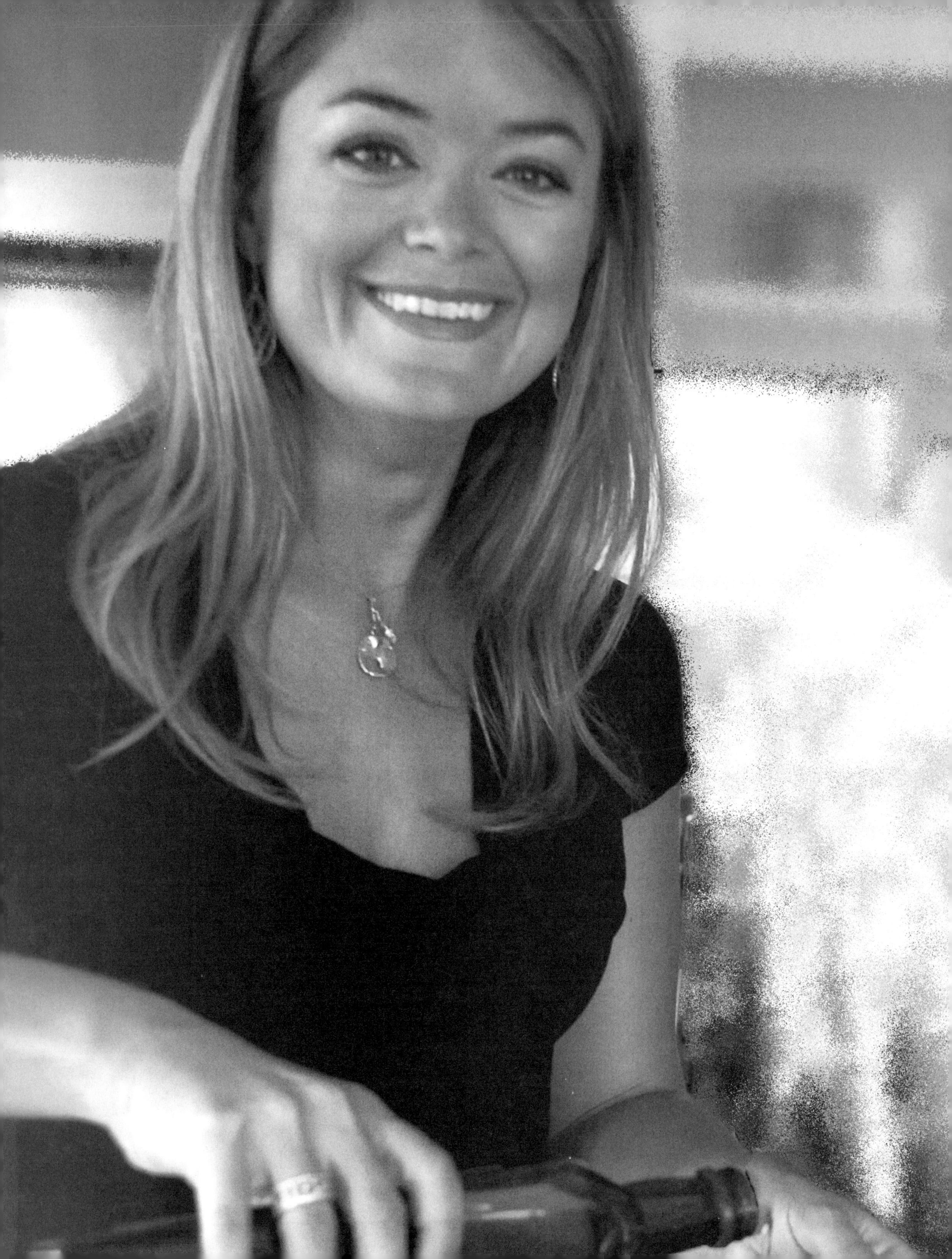

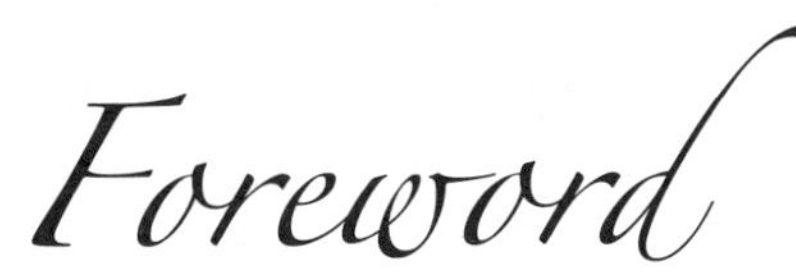

Foreword

Creating a labor of love can resemble the process of bringing a child into being. Such is the case with *Cooking for Fertility – Foods to Nourish Your Fertile Soul*. The idea arose at a Fertile Soul retreat when Kathryn Simmons Flynn and I were discussing how we could get her magnificent Cooking for Fertility work out in the world. We had been compiling recipes and eating plans for quite a while, but it appeared that birthing a book was what needed to happen next. Fast forward a couple of years, a few edits, life changes, and Braxton Hicks contractions later: and like any mother being used in the grand universal timing to bring forth life, she persevered. Kathryn has been treating women's health through better nutrition in The Fertile Soul's advisory program for years, and I hear over and over again: "When is she going to publish a cookbook?"

Well, the time has finally come. Although I may honor myself by saying I played midwife to this project, what I've really done is to watch Kathryn research, love, nurture, and now bring into emergence this exciting, new book. I am proud to have been a small part of it. And I can guarantee you – it's been worth the wait.

Based on a firm foundation of utilizing whole foods that nourish one's reproductive system and feed the soul, Kathryn has been able to make the concept of relying on certain foods to rectify patterns of imbalance into an easy to use, indispensable kitchen tool. Most of us, including the medical profession, have strayed from healthy remedies that nature intended. A Chinese proverb cautions us,

Those who take medicine and neglect their diet waste the skills of the physician.

Yet, a sound eating plan doesn't defy conventional treatment; even the "father of medicine," Hippocrates, recognized,

Let food be thy medicine and medicine be thy food.

Imagine that eating according to simple guidelines, following easy to understand recipes, and indulging in a gourmet-eating plan can bring you closer to better health, greater fertility, and the sheer enjoyment of eating well. We insist that your fertility eating plan not be one of drudgery and deprivation. It must feed your soul, delight your senses, and bring you into the flow of life.

My greatest hope is that this book can bring you into better reproductive health, provide a sound eating plan throughout your pregnancy, and help your child develop healthy nutritional patterns even before she has taken her first bite of food.

Enjoy this process. You must become a vessel for yourself before you can become a vessel for another.

With gratitude and love,

Randine Lewis

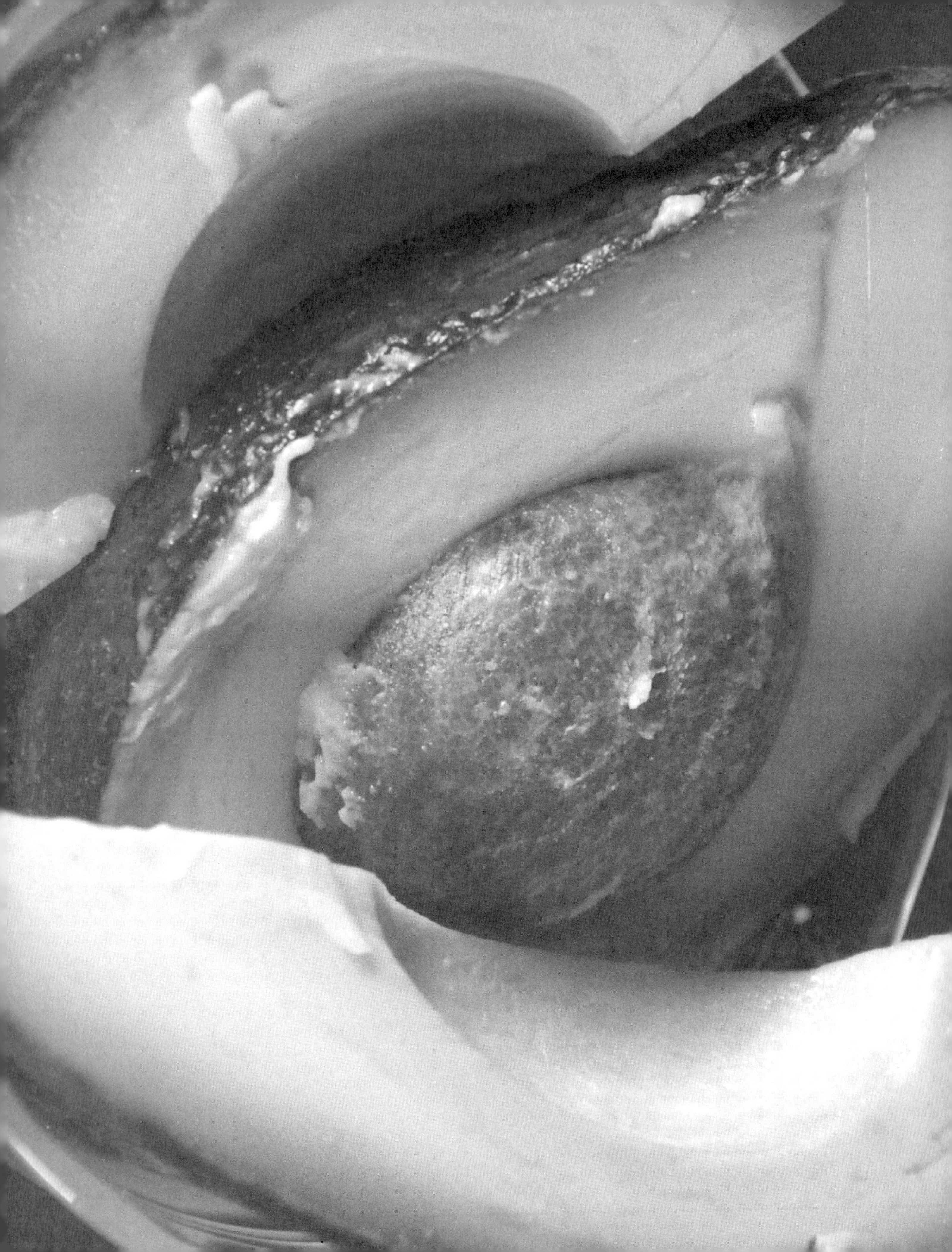

Eating for Fertility

"The doctor of the future will give no medicines, but will interest his patients in the care of the human frame, in diet, and in the causes of disease."
– *Thomas Edison*

In the Western world one in five couples has difficulty conceiving a child. Their sub-fertility often results from less than optimal health. Our bodies carry deep evolutionary wisdom, including innate protective mechanisms that can safeguard our own health and that of future generations by not allowing us to conceive until we are in good health.

Endometriosis, ovarian failure, poor quality eggs, recurrent miscarriage and other degenerative diseases and causes of poor reproductive health have become widespread. In many cases, they result from our cells not getting the nutrition they require. Our bodies cannot cope with the high amounts of processed and refined foods, environmental toxins, and persistent stress in our lives. We are part of nature, yet our way of living is far from what nature intends.

More and more studies show that good nutrition and healthy life habits can increase conception rates. Beyond assisting fertility, healthful lifestyle practices can also prevent and heal disease. When our body systems don't work as efficiently as they could, one of the best ways to support their highest function is to nourish them.

For thousands of years, Traditional Chinese Medicine (TCM) has used dietary therapy to correct imbalances and support hormonal and reproductive harmony and overall wellness. Sun Si-miao, a famous doctor of Chinese medicine, believed the most important therapy was regulating a patient's diet. Dietary therapy could then be enhanced with acupuncture and herbal treatment.

Chinese medicine considers the ability to bring forth life to be a woman's natural state from the time of menarche until she reaches menopause. Sub-fertility results from imbalances within the network of organs, hormones and energy systems within a woman's body; recent studies and thousands of years of experience have demonstrated that many of these imbalances are correctable.

Cooking for Fertility – Foods to Nourish Your Fertile Soul introduces you to the wisdom of TCM Dietary Therapy as it applies to restoring and replenishing your reproductive capacity. It provides general recommendations at the beginning of each section and specific information about the impact of particular ingredients preceding each recipe. This book is a guide for using delicious whole foods to nourish your body to correct internal imbalances and to create a healthy internal environment conducive to conceiving and carrying a healthy baby.

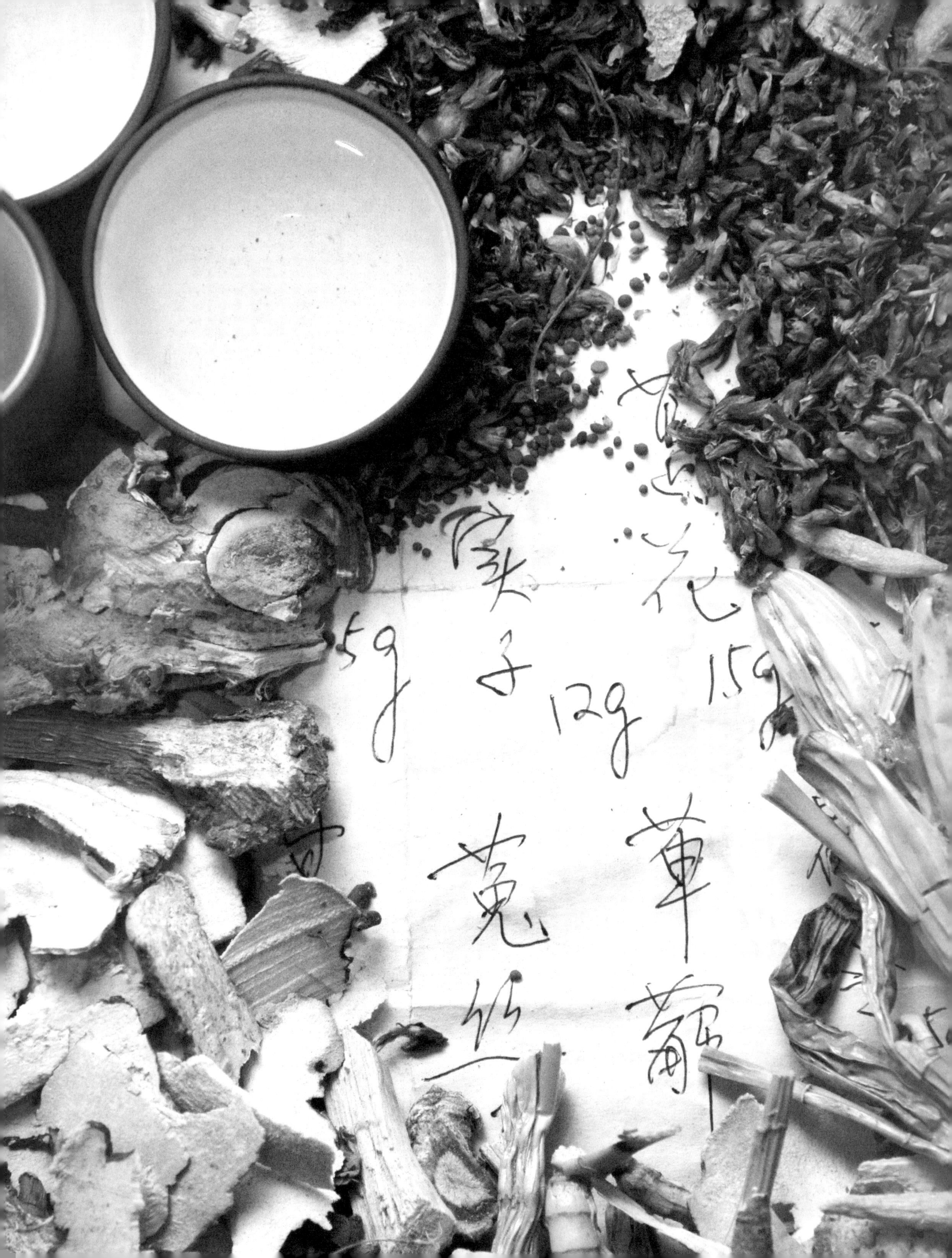

15g
12g
5g
萆薢

Chinese Medicine and the Reproductive System

Chinese medicine views the body as a microcosm of nature itself: a complex energetic system comprised of two major divisions – yin (cool, moist, receptive) and yang (warm, dynamic, active) that must be in balance for health to result. We also embody three "treasures" – essence, energy, and spirit – that must be in harmony; four substances – qi, blood, fluid, and jing; and five interactive energies – water, wood, fire, earth and metal – that govern the organ and energetic systems (kidney, liver, heart, spleen-pancreas, and lungs). Traditional Chinese medicine seeks to restore harmony in the interactions of these energetic systems so that pathology (in the form of dampness, phlegm, dryness, heat, cold, exterior pathogens, interior factors, deficient conditions, and excess conditions such as blood stasis and qi stagnation) does not result. When the body is imbalanced, disease is likely to result. When we can identify patterns tending toward imbalance, we can prevent many disease states. Dietary intervention is one of the first courses of action to help restore the body's harmonious energetic state.

THE KIDNEY SYSTEM

The Kidney system governs reproductive and urinary functions, internal secretions, hormone production, the central nervous system, and the process of growth, development, maturation and decline. The Kidney system is the root of all organ systems, and its health impacts on and is impacted not only by our physical being, but also our mind, emotions, spirit, and our essential nature. Nourishing our Kidney "essence" is essential to supporting our inherent fertility. Each of us is born with a finite amount of life "essence", which is referred to in Chinese medicine as *congenital jing*. Congenital jing fuels our life's journey; it is a finite resource. As we deplete our congenital jing, we can replenish our essence reserves by accumulating new jing by making conscious diet and lifestyle choices. Building jing with diet involves choosing foods that promote the strengthening and development of the body and mind. Such foods also provide renewal, longevity, reproductive capacity and protection from premature aging[1].

LIFESTYLE HABITS THAT DRAIN FERTILITY

In our modern world, we have many habits that drain our jing and negatively impact our fertility. The most common cause of Kidney Deficiency is physical and mental overwork. Multiple pregnancies, miscarriages, and childbirth also deplete Kidney Essence in women. Taxing to the reproductive system of both women and men are:

- Work stress

- Long work hours
- Excessive cerebral activity without physical release
- Mental anxiety
- Lack of relaxation
- Inadequate sleep
- Hurried, irregular eating schedules
- Stimulants like caffeine, drugs and alcohol
- Excessive sexual activity
- Hormonal stimulation

Address these issues by simply slowing down and making deliberate diet and lifestyle changes to replenish your system. As you begin practicing moderation in more areas of your life, getting adequate rest, daily exercise and proper cellular nutrition, you nourish yourself from the inside out. You feel more in harmony with the natural flow of life and processes that govern your fertility.

Digestion and Reproduction

"The human body begins its development in a saline solution in the womb and is nourished and cleansed by blood that has almost the same composition as sea water"[2].

The reproductive organs, which correspond to the Water element in Chinese medicine, favor cooked foods, especially those simmered slowly in liquid (soups, stews, beans and legumes). The corresponding flavor of the water element is salt, which is preferably ingested by adding the beneficial minerals from seaweed to soups, stews and casseroles. When eating to support fertility, consume a mostly alkaline diet of vegetables, fruits, and sea vegetables, and limit acidic foods including alcohol, sugar, excess animal protein, wheat and dairy.

THE ROLE OF THE SPLEEN-PANCREAS IN DIGESTION AND REPRODUCTION

TCM considers the spleen, stomach and pancreas an interactive unit of food intake, utilization and distribution. Because of the Spleen-Pancreas' primary role in the digestion, transformation and distribution of nutrients, our "Spleen Qi Diet" uses basic principles that nourish and support the Spleen to enhance reproductive function.

According to Traditional Chinese Medicine, the Spleen-Pancreas extracts and collects nutrients from food, breaks them down, and transforms them into essential metabolic processes. Your digestive system must be functioning optimally for cellular and endocrine health. When digestive function is strong, the reproductive hormones, produced by the Kidneys and metabolized by the Liver, function more efficiently.

In addition to digestion, the Spleen-Pancreas system governs metabolism, blood production, immune regulation, and thyroid function. As the physical Spleen-Pancreas system breaks down and transforms food, its mental system governs breaking the world down into digestible thought processes. When the physical Spleen is not operating efficiently, our digestion can become clogged. When the mind aspect of the Spleen system is not functioning optimally, our thoughts can become repetitive and worrisome – resulting in more digestive and psychological obstructions.

By following the principles of the Spleen Qi Diet you will experience:

- Enhanced reproductive capability
- Increased energy, improved digestion
- Stabilized hormones and mood
- Clarity of Intention and body—mind connection
- Your ideal healthy weight (BMI)

Because of the Spleen system's crucial role in metabolic processing, all recipes will follow Spleen Qi dietary guidelines, and will be modified to restore balance in all energetic systems necessary for a healthy functioning reproductive system. For a more detailed understanding of Chinese medicine and fertility as well as the Chinese medicine diagnoses referred to throughout this book, please see *The Infertility Cure* by Randine Lewis.

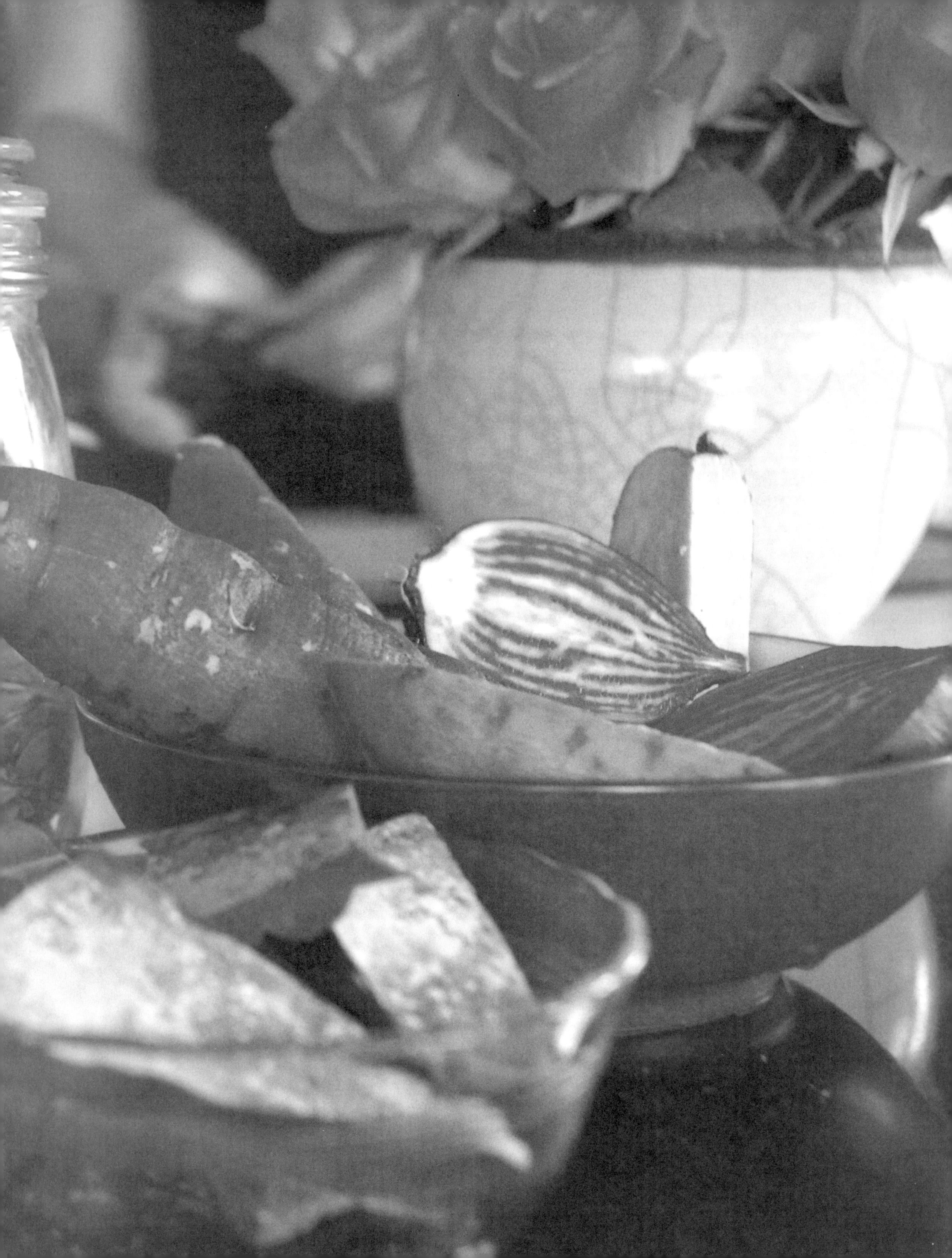

Basic Guidelines

Cooking for Fertility: Foods to Nourish Your Fertile Soul *will introduce the Spleen Qi Diet with general recommendations and lifestyle practices, which help ensure optimal intake of nutrients, digestion and distribution to the reproductive and other organ systems. See these guidelines as an opportunity rather than as a restriction (and thus, another source of stress). Becoming more aware of the choices you are making and exploring new foods you are less familiar with can bring great joy as you discover new tastes and feel your health improving and energy increasing.*

As you become more familiar with eating in accordance with the diet's basic guidelines, you can begin to further supplement your diet with foods that are healing for you personally based on your individual diagnosis and tendencies. Cooking for Fertility *provides guidance on customizing your diet in the lifestyle and meal plan recommendations in the appendix.*

1. Replace refined carbohydrates and wheat

Wheat is one of the eight most common allergens. It encourages growth of unhealthy bacteria, which impedes digestion and absorption of nutrients. When enhancing fertility and to support the Spleen, we want to ensure that nutrients are being distributed optimally to support reproductive function. Unsprouted wheat and refined carbohydrates (foods that have been processed and stripped of vital nutrients including B vitamins, fiber and iron) contain sugar-binding proteins called Lectins that adhere to the cells, causing the blood to agglutinate (form clots). This creates internal inflammatory reactions, impeding the hormonal system, causing food sensitivities, allergies and autoimmune reactions.

Symptoms of wheat sensitivity include: bloating, gas, constipation, irritability, depression, fatigue, and the aggravation of common diseases including arthritis, psoriasis and eczema. Many people notice significant improvements in their health and well-being after removing wheat from their diet.

It is important to note that having wheat sensitivity is different than being diagnosed with gluten intolerance. Celiac disease, an allergy or intolerance to gluten, is a chronic intestinal disorder in which nutrients cannot be absorbed. If you decide to abstain from gluten, simply replace spelt and oats with any of the other gluten-free grains listed in the Fertile Soul Pantry section. When shopping, it should be safe to purchase products marked as gluten-free, as you are assured they will not contain wheat.

2. Choose whole fat goat or sheep dairy over cow dairy

A recent study released by Harvard Medical School, The Nurses Health Study, show that women who consume low-fat dairy are more likely to have difficulty conceiving than women who consume whole-fat dairy. The Nurses Study claims that whole milk and ice cream are the most potent fertility foods.[3] The Fertile Soul also advocates consuming whole-fat foods to support conception – however, we recommend avoiding ice cream except as a special treat because of its dampening effect on digestion, which slows the distribution of nutrients.

Our milk of choice is whole-fat goat dairy. Goat dairy has a less complex protein structure than cow dairy, making it far easier to digest. The calcium in milk is bound to the protein cassein, which is difficult to break down. Don't worry about calcium levels – calcium is much more bioavailable from other sources such as bok choy, broccoli, almonds, and from sources such as oyster shell, coral calcium, and colloidal minerals.

Soy milk has become a very popular alternative that we recommend enjoying in limited quantities. Due to the "soy craze" that has occurred over the past 10 years, soy is appearing in many products of which we may not even be aware. Since excess soy consumption can interfere with natural estrogen receptors, we recommend avoiding soy isolate proteins in bars and shakes. You may consume soy in its unrefined form from sources like tempeh and edamame.

To address dairy sensitivities and for the benefits of a more varied diet, please consider such delicious substitutes as hemp milk and almond milk.

3. Substitute refined sugars and artificial sweeteners with natural low-glycemic replacements

High-glycemic foods activate the pancreatic system, interfering with the efficient production and utilization of the reproductive hormones. When we consume anything with fast, blood sugar-raising effects – like fruit juice and refined carbohydrates – the blood sugar rises, insulin is released to handle the sugar, and the blood sugar later plummets. In response to the continual fluctuations in blood sugar levels, the body releases stress hormones to equalize blood sugar levels and maintain homeostasis. In the resulting milieu of glucose, insulin, and adrenocortical hormones, the reproductive hormones move out of the way, and the tissues actually stop responding to estrogen and progesterone while the stress hormones dominate. When we continually subject our systems to this endocrine storm, the body remains poised to "fight or flight"; and until the internal stressor passes, it literally cannot settle down into "feed and breed" mode, where it can respond adequately to the presence of reproductive hormones.

Fortunately, we can recondition the body by removing high-glycemic foods. To learn how to use low-glycemic sweeteners like agave nectar, please see the Indulge section. To maintain steady blood sugar and energy levels, eat small meals with balanced protein and carbohydrates throughout the day and drink adequate amounts of water to stay hydrated.

It is particularly important to avoid soda pop, which contains harmful chemicals like high-fructose corn syrup and Aspartame. In a study by Madelon Price, Aspartame consumption was shown to create infertility in rodents. She specifically noted that aspartame disrupts the release of prolactin, luteinizing hormone and growth hormone, all of which govern sexual function. Aspartame at both low and high doses impact the pituitary gland, resulting in abnormal releases of hormones and ultimately disrupting the neurons responsible for transmission.[4] Try sparkling water with a splash of juice as a soda alternative or kombucha tea, with its many healing benefits (more in the Hydrate section).

4. Eliminate coffee and excess caffeine

Both caffeinated and decaffeinated coffee contain volatile oils that congest the Liver, activate the adrenal hormones and fuel the stress response that impairs reproductive capacity. These oils and their effect are a bigger concern than caffeine. Sensitive individuals can still feel this adrenaline jolt with a cup of decaf.

Try replacing the coffee in your diet with non-caffeinated herbal teas – see the Hydrate section for information on their healing benefits. If you are prone to anxiety and stress, even slight amounts of caffeine such as those that are in green tea can exacerbate these conditions.

If you are not sensitive to caffeine but need to wean yourself from coffee, explore the benefits of green tea, which beneficially dilates blood vessels (coffee has the opposite effect, incidentally, constricting them). Green tea has been the "antioxidant" of choice used by the Chinese for more than 4,000 years to cure ailments from headaches to depression.

When you become pregnant it is important to cut out caffeine altogether. A recent study by Kaiser Permanente found that ingesting the equivalent of two cups of caffeine boosts your chance of miscarriage. It also notes that the source of the caffeine is insignificant and can be "coffee, soda, tea or hot chocolate." Dr. De-Kun Li, the study's lead author, confirms that: "caffeine is dangerous during pregnancy because it can cross through the placenta to the fetus and it can be difficult for the fetus to metabolize the caffeine. Caffeine may influence cell development and decrease blood flow to the placenta."[5]

5. Avoid alcohol, nicotine and drugs

Alcohol, nicotine, caffeine, drugs and unnecessary over the counter medications should be avoided whenever possible. All of these substances agitate the system and drain our essence at an accelerated rate. Excessive use interferes with energetic Liver functions like storing the blood and directing it to the uterus, governing the release of ovulatory hormones, and regulating the menstrual cycle. We recommend that women who are trying to conceive remove alcohol from their diet altogether, especially if they have a tendency toward Liver Qi Stagnation (symptoms include ovulatory breast pain, premenstrual tension, irritability, and headaches), or Excess Heat (symptoms include fevers, night sweats, hot flashes, and hot skin irritations such as rashes, herpes and acne).

6. Limit raw foods and avoid cold food and beverages

The Spleen system functions better at warm temperatures. Cooking assists with breaking food down, facilitating the digestion process and enabling the body to absorb more nutrients. Although raw food diets have many health benefits, particularly in terms of radical detoxification, in supporting fertility, our goal is to replenish and nourish fertility while gently releasing excess toxins where required.

As a general rule, lightly cooked foods build Qi and contribute to an overall sense of grounding, while raw foods are detoxifying and have a tendency to activate the mind.

Visualize the Spleen as a cooking pot that performs optimally when kept at room temperature to keep digestive fires burning. Not only do cold and damp foods put out the digestive fire: The body actually expends heat and energy trying to absorb nutrients, which starves the other organs of greater nourishment. Ice cream is a big offender with its ice-cold, "damp" properties: It not only puts out the fire, but can also create a sludge effect that impedes digestion. Drinking with meals – particularly iced drinks – also puts out the digestive fire and forces the body to work even harder to break down food. Try to chew each bite 30 times to liquefy food and activate digestive enzymes in the mouth that assist in the transformation of nutrients to a form the body can absorb. The combination of digestive enzymes and saliva produced by chewing also prevents the Chinese medicine condition of Dryness, another condition that slows digestive processes.

7. Choose organic seasonal foods

Selecting seasonal, fresh organic ingredients brings you as close to the earth as possible to optimally nourish your body. Ideally, we would buy fresh food each day and cook it each night for the greatest amount of food energy. If your lifestyle permits, buy from a local farmers' market or other source of locally grown produce.

In this day and age, the typical diet includes a lot of refined carbohydrates, antibiotics, hormone-infused meat and milk, trans fats, excess starch and canned produce. Many fertility impairments – hormonal imbalances, endometriosis, polycystic ovaries, fibroids, and others – are due to "estrogen dominance."

Rather than turning to medications, we can override estrogen dominance by consuming more plant phytoestrogens, which are found in products such as soybeans, edamame and tofu. Natural phytoestrogens beneficially replace the harmful xenoestrogens from the estrogen receptor sites on our cells. The important thing to note is that these protective properties are found in whole-food sources, not in concentrated soy products or isolated pills and powders.

Cruciferous vegetables (such as broccoli and cauliflower) contain di-indolymethane (DIM), a compound that stimulates more efficient use of estrogen by increasing the liver's ability to metabolize estradiol. If organic produce is not readily available to you, soak your fruits and vegetables in 2 teaspoons salt, 1/4 cup of vinegar and a quart of cold water for 10 minutes to remove unwanted pesticides and critters. As much as possible, choose fresh organic fruits and vegetables and hormone-free organic meats.

8. Model your diet on an Asian diet

When eating for fertility, model an Asian diet. Visualize a plate filled mostly with steamed vegetables, some whole grains such as brown rice, and a palm-sized portion of protein. As a general guideline, consume up to 4 oz. of animal protein per day or 4-10 oz. of plant protein (nuts, beans and legumes). The rest of your diet should include lots of vegetables, fruits, wheat-free grains and healthy fats.

By consuming a balanced protein and carbohydrate at each meal and snack, you stabilize energy and blood sugar levels throughout the day. We recommend 40-50% of your calories come from complex carbohydrates, 20-30% from protein and 30% from unsaturated fats. In those with insulin resistance or glucose intolerance, a higher (40%) protein content may be required.

What about high-protein diets?

"Low-carbohydrate, high-protein eating plans have well-known side effects: Over 30 years of research studies, all concur that high protein consumption greatly puts one at risk for bone loss and kidney failure."[6] Cutting out carbohydrates, as recommended by diets like Atkins, helped many people to lose weight initially, but the results are not sustainable. High-protein diets most often lead to cravings for simple carbohydrates (white flours, sugars, candy and alcohol) that spike blood sugar and disrupt insulin function. Additional side effects that result from too much protein are: nausea, fatigue, bad breath, constipation, muscle cramps, headaches, aggression, and irritability. Low-carbohydrate diets also weaken immunity, cell regeneration and brain function. In one study conducted in mice, carbohydrate consumption was limited and their embryos were unable to implant. For optimum health, eat adequate amounts of complex carbohydrates from whole, organic fruits and vegetables.

The importance of grains

Whole grains contain glyconutrients or sugar chains, which help to re-harmonize the body's taste buds while curbing intense sugar cravings and providing the following benefits:

1. Coat and protect all body cells against viruses
2. Regulate immune response
3. Are anti-inflammatory
4. Support neurotransmitter function in the brain[7]

Glyconutrients also are plentiful in vegetables, nuts and algae. The Chinese eat 30% more grains than Americans and have significantly better health rates, including lower incidence of breast cancer and heart disease.[8] The typical American diet includes too many of the wrong types of grains, such as white flour, pasta, bread, rolls, crackers and refined carbohydrates.

9. Include good sources of healthy fats

In the Nurses Study done by Harvard Medical School, trans fats were proven to negatively impact fertility, even at the low rate of two per cent of daily calories or four grams, the equivalent amount "in two tablespoons of stick margarine, one medium order of fast-food French fries, or one doughnut."[9]

It is also well known in the medical community that cholesterol is necessary for hormone production, and that fat cells store hormones. Women who do not consume enough good fats or have enough body fat often suffer from irregular cycles or lose their menses completely. Thus, eating good fats supports fertility.

Healthy oils and fats:

Organic, unrefined oils for cooking: extra virgin olive oil, sesame oil and high-oleic sunflower oil.

Omega and GLA (Gamma Linolenic Acid) oils have countless health benefits. They help to heal the Liver and Gall bladder, have anti-inflammatory and anticlotting properties, reduce symptoms of PMS, depressive mood swings and other degenerative diseases. Drizzle the following oils on breakfast cereals and steamed vegetables: Usana-brand Optomega, flax oil, evening primrose oil, borage oil, black currant oil, pumpkin seed oil and chia seed oil.

Healthy fat food sources:

Omega 3 fatty acids: salmon, sardines, mackerel, flax seeds, chia seed, walnuts, pumpkin seeds, and dark leafy greens.[10]

Monounsaturated fats: almonds, coconut, olives, walnuts, sunflower seeds and avocadoes.[11]

10. Reduce stress

"To keep the body in good health is a duty.
Otherwise we shall not be able to keep our minds strong and clear."

- *Buddha*

Before we were born our adrenal glands, kidneys and reproductive organs developed together. The adrenal gland dominates this triad, suppressing the proper functioning of the kidney and ovaries when fear is present. Although fear ensures self-preservation and survival, persistent, irrational fear indicates a Kidney imbalance. When we fuel fear with daily stressors, it can become pathological, disrupting all body functions. Extremes of the emotions of fear and stress can also cause severe hormonal fluctuations in any endocrine organ, upsetting our reproductive capacity. The adrenal-kidney-ovarian triad governs the deepest aspect of our being – the governing, penetrating and conception meridians where our fertility and creativity arise.

It is common knowledge that stress is a predicator of disease. Studies show that women who function at high stress levels are over 90 per cent less likely to conceive. Animals in the wild do not go into heat when they are under stress. But we human creatures try to override nature and conceive anyway without changing our lifestyle. Trying to force a pregnancy when an imbalanced body is not ready causes it to raise even more protective mechanisms to prevent conception. Stress hormones like cortisol are released by the adrenals into the bloodstream, signaling the body to prepare for "fight or flight;" the body responds by sending blood only to those organs necessary to sustain life, while minimizing the circulation to the reproductive organs. This state of stress may disrupts the levels of reproductive hormones such as elevated prolactin, high FSH (Follicle-stimulating hormone), low progesterone, high estradiol, potentially causing a lack of menstruation, anovulation, poor uterine lining, or even a diagnosis of unexplained infertility. Minimizing stress by slowing down the pace of your lifestyle with awareness practices, exercise routines and adequate rest, complemented by eliminating external toxins such as alcohol, refined foods, caffeine, nicotine, drugs and non-essential medication, can help to eliminate a lot of the body's stress and preserve your essence.

11. Create "YOU TIME"

Dr. Robin Tiberi believes that "female fertility is about developing the female principle of yin receptivity. Yin receptivity is openness and allowing."[11a] When we take time for ourselves, we feel grounded, calm and able to respond to life's stressors. When we are drained, we may feel scattered, further activating our stress hormones and exacerbating burnout. Activities that promote a sense of relaxation and calm replenish our systems, which are often over-taxed by the emphasis in our outward world (yang) at the expense of our inner world (yin). It is believed that we now process more information in one day than our ancestors did in one year. This immense stress takes its toll on our poor, overworked bodyminds.

All productive fields require fallow time in which to regenerate. In Chinese medicine, the season of winter is associated with the water element (kidneys, reproductive organs and adrenals). Winter is known as the time of hibernation and replenishment. It is also, notably, the time of increased sperm production. To live in accordance with our authentic self and in greatest health, we must practice greater awareness of our most basic needs: What is my body is asking for? Food? Rest? Water? Quiet time? Meditation? What best supports my unique make-up and gives me the foundation to meet life's demands? In Chinese medicine, the reproductive system also corresponds to the ears. When we go within ourselves, become still and hear our inner voice, we begin to make decisions that support our very foundation.

Stress-reducing techniques to replenish your deepest reserves

- Quiet reflection
- Qi Gong
- Deep belly breathing
- Meditation
- Visualization
- Listening to meditative music
- A bath in Epson salts or Lavender Oil
- Journaling
- Adequate rest
- Massage
- Acupuncture

12. Get exercise and movement each day

Though many of us have grown up in a culture of exercise with a "no pain no gain" attitude, the journey of fertility requires a different outlook. The goal is to find exercises you enjoy that replenish your energy reserves while you circulate fresh blood and oxygen to your organs, flood the body with feel-good endorphins, support digestion and maintain a healthy weight.

Some of our favorite exercises for fertility:

- Walking
- Yoga
- Swimming
- Qi Gong
- Gardening
- Dancing

13. Mindful Eating: Pleasure and Food

"What you eat impacts your fertility as much as what you think about what you eat"

- *Randine Lewis*

It has been said that the energy we infuse our food with is the energy that enters our body. If we are hurried and rushed while we are cooking, this is how we may feel when we eat, which may in turn effect our digestion. Do what you can to enjoy the entire cooking process and even turn it into a calming meditation.

Consider the following experience: set the table for yourself, put on some calming music and light some candles. Take some time to be grateful for the food on your plate and the blessings in your life to infuse you with the feelings of love and appreciation, and invoke pleasure. Silent or out loud, a blessing can set the tone for a delicious meal. Now that you are set to enjoy your meal, take the time to taste the food. Slow down your eating by aiming for 20-30 chews per bite, putting your fork down in between. It takes at least 20 minutes to activate the signals that you feel full, so prolonging your meal will help you avoid overeating.

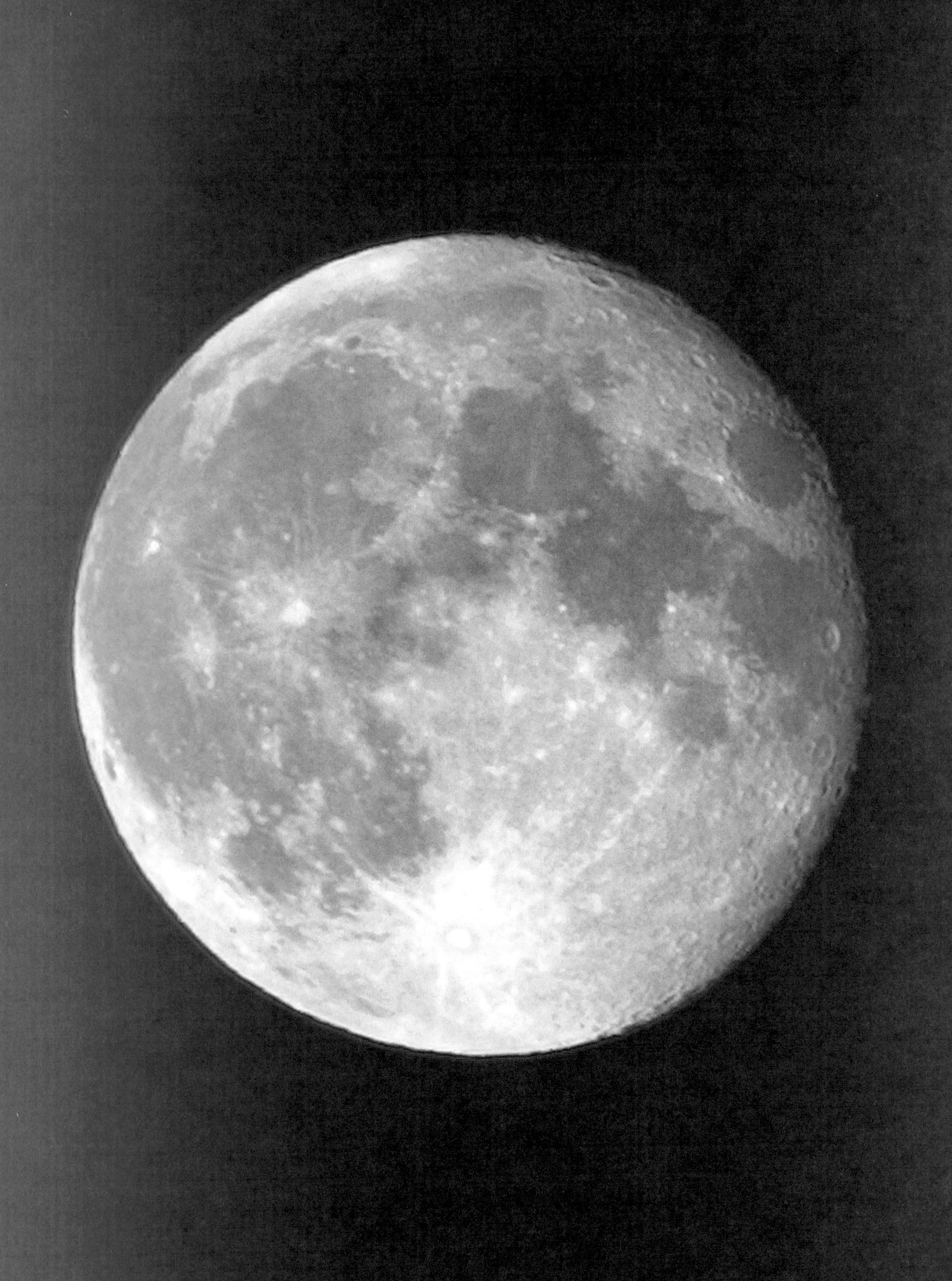

Aligning with the Cycles of the Moon

Above all else, enjoy your food. Learn healthy eating practices, but don't deprive yourself. Love your body and what you put into it.

Chinese medicine likens the menstrual cycle to the four phases of the moon: follicular (waxing), ovulatory (full), luteal (waning), and menses (dark or new moon). Like the moon cycle, a typical cycle lasts 28-30 days and has 3-5 days of flowing red blood. By taking a closer look at your individual symptoms, you can identify areas of imbalance and use dietary therapy to harmonize and regulate your flow. In addition to the general guidelines provided here, the appendix includes additional lifestyle guidelines and meal plans for common patterns of imbalance.

Follicular phase

The follicular phase is more "Yin" in nature – receptive, growing, deep, and cooling – an important time to practice introspection and build up your reserves. During this stage, your body nourishes the follicles that house the eggs, and produces more estrogen, a Yin fluid that "generates a plush uterine lining, causes cervical changes and produces fertile cervical mucus during ovulation. At this time, the body prepares the cave of the Uterus to accept the fertilized egg and nurture the evolving embryo."[12]

If your body is deficient in Yin energies, you may be prone to any or all of the following symptoms: short cycles, scant cervical mucus, vaginal dryness, night sweats, hot flashes and back or knee weakness. To resolve them, incorporate cooling foods such as apples, asparagus, bananas, barley, bean sprouts, beets, blackberries, bulgur, cheese, chlorella, chickpeas, clams, crab, cuttlefish, duck, eggplant, eggs, honey, grapes, kidney beans, jellyfish, lemon, malt, mango, melon, milk, mulberries, organ meats, oysters, peas, pears, pineapples, pomegranate, pork, rabbit, raspberries, rice, seaweed, shellfish, soybeans, spirulina, string beans, tofu, tomato, watermelon, yams.

The follicular phase is also the time to nourish blood, which feeds the growing egg, and nourishes the endometrial lining.

If you are experiencing symptoms of Blood Deficiency – scant menstrual blood, amenorrhea, premenstrual dizziness, hair loss, and dry skin – the following foods can help nourish the blood: Aduki bean, apricot, beef, beetroot, blackberries, bone marrow, eggs, cuttlefish, dark leafy greens, date, dandelion, fig, grape, kidney bean, liver, hormone-free meat and liver, microalgae, nettle, octopus, oyster, parsley, raspberry, sardine, spinach, spirulina, sweet rice and watercress.

Ovulatory Phase

The ovulatory phase, like the full moon, is a dynamic time where the results of the follicular phase are realized. If yin and blood have adequately reached their peak, the process of ovulation will be smooth. When our energy stagnates, the ovulatory phase can be weak, insufficient, or sluggish, resulting in symptoms like ovulatory breast tenderness, a dull ache in the lower abdomen, prolonged LH (luteinizing hormone) surge, stair-stepped basal body temperature charts, and general irritability during ovulation.

Foods that can help resolve this stagnant energy include: Basil, caraway, cardamom, carrot, cayenne, chive, clove, coriander, dill seed, garlic, marjoram, mustard leaf, orange peel, peppermint, radish, rosemary, spearmint, star anise, tangerine peel, thyme, and turmeric.

Luteal Phase

During the luteal phase your body produces progesterone, a Kidney yang energy that has an expanding, invigorating, and warming momentum. Progesterone is "a hormone secreted by the corpus luteum of the ovary after ovulation" and is responsible for "transform[ing] the endometrial tissue so it can hold a fertilized ovum."[13] If you are Kidney yang deficient you may be experiencing premenstrual low back pain, low libido, nighttime urination, and general coldness in nature. To resolve Kidney yang deficiency include warming foods such as anchovies, aduki beans, anise, basil, beets, black beans, black pepper, caraway, cayenne, cherries, chestnut, chicken, chives, cinnamon bark, cloves, coriander, cumin, dates, dill, fennel, fenugreek seed, garlic, dried ginger, kidney, lamb, leeks, lentils, lobster, mussels, mustard leaf, mutton, nutmeg, oats, onions, peach, pine nuts, pistachio, quinoa, raspberry, rosemary, sage, scallions, shrimp, spelt, star anise, sweet brown rice, thyme, trout, turnip, walnuts.

When the cycle wanes at the end of the luteal phase, if an embryo has not notified the body of its presence, we prepare for the dark of the moon, the return of the energies to the center of the body to begin a new cycle.

The Liver is important in reproduction and menstruation due to its role in directing menstruation and hormones. During the premenstrual period the Liver shifts the Blood flow from other body parts to the Uterus. Right before menstruation, when the Liver is busy directing the body to menstruate, it has a tendency to neglect its other functions of keeping the Qi (energy) and emotions flowing smoothly. If the channels remain blocked, the flow of energy to the Uterus will be impeded, and the menses are associated with pain and cramping.

When the Liver system is not functioning smoothly, the hormonal system is not either. The Uterus itself can become a toxic environment, hostile to implantation. Excess hormones, including estrogen, that are not metabolized effectively can build up, causing stagnation due to the liver's inability to adequately process hormones. [Leafy green vegetables contain DIM (di-indolymethane), which help metabolize excess estrogen.]

If you experience any or all of the following symptoms of Liver Qi Stagnation – premenstrual symptoms, depression, anger, sadness, weepiness headaches, breast pain, cramps, irritability, headaches, migraines, breast tenderness at ovulation – you may want to include the foods that we suggested to move energy during the ovulatory transition.

Menstruation and the Quality of the Blood flow

The Chinese concept of the Heart encompasses the aspect of mind and spirit as well as governing the Blood and circulatory system. The heart provides Blood for the Uterus; the Uterine Vessel, called the Bao Mai, links the Heart and the Uterus. The Su Wen (a Chinese medical classic) says: "The Uterine Vessel pertains to the Heart and extends to the Uterus," and "when the period does not come it means the Uterine Vessel is obstructed." Signs of uterine vessel obstruction and uterine blood stagnation are indicated by lack of menstrual bleeding, dark, brown or black menstrual blood, clotting during the period, fibroids, or endometriosis.

The following foods can help resolve blood stasis: abalone, beets, bilberry, Brussels sprouts, chestnuts, chili pepper, chives, crab, cucumbers, dark green vegetables, eggplant, evening primrose oil, fish and fish oil, hawthorn berries, kelp, lemons, limes, linseed oil, mustard leaf, nuts and seed oils, onion, peaches, saffron, scallions, seaweed, spirulina, squid, sturgeon, turnips, and vinegar.

In the absence of blood stagnation, the body's energies have a natural tendency to go within during the bleeding or dark of the moon phase. Warming, nourishing foods can help harmonize this phase. We encourage soups, root vegetables and yang-tonifying foods that help support the late luteal phase. This is also the time to allow your body to detoxify with whole fruits, vegetables, and broths. (Harsh detoxifying plans are not recommend during the active phase of the cycle when implantation may have occurred.) To resolve the symptoms listed above and strengthen your fertility, modify your diet to ensure that each organ system is getting the nutrients it needs to support its reproductive tasks.

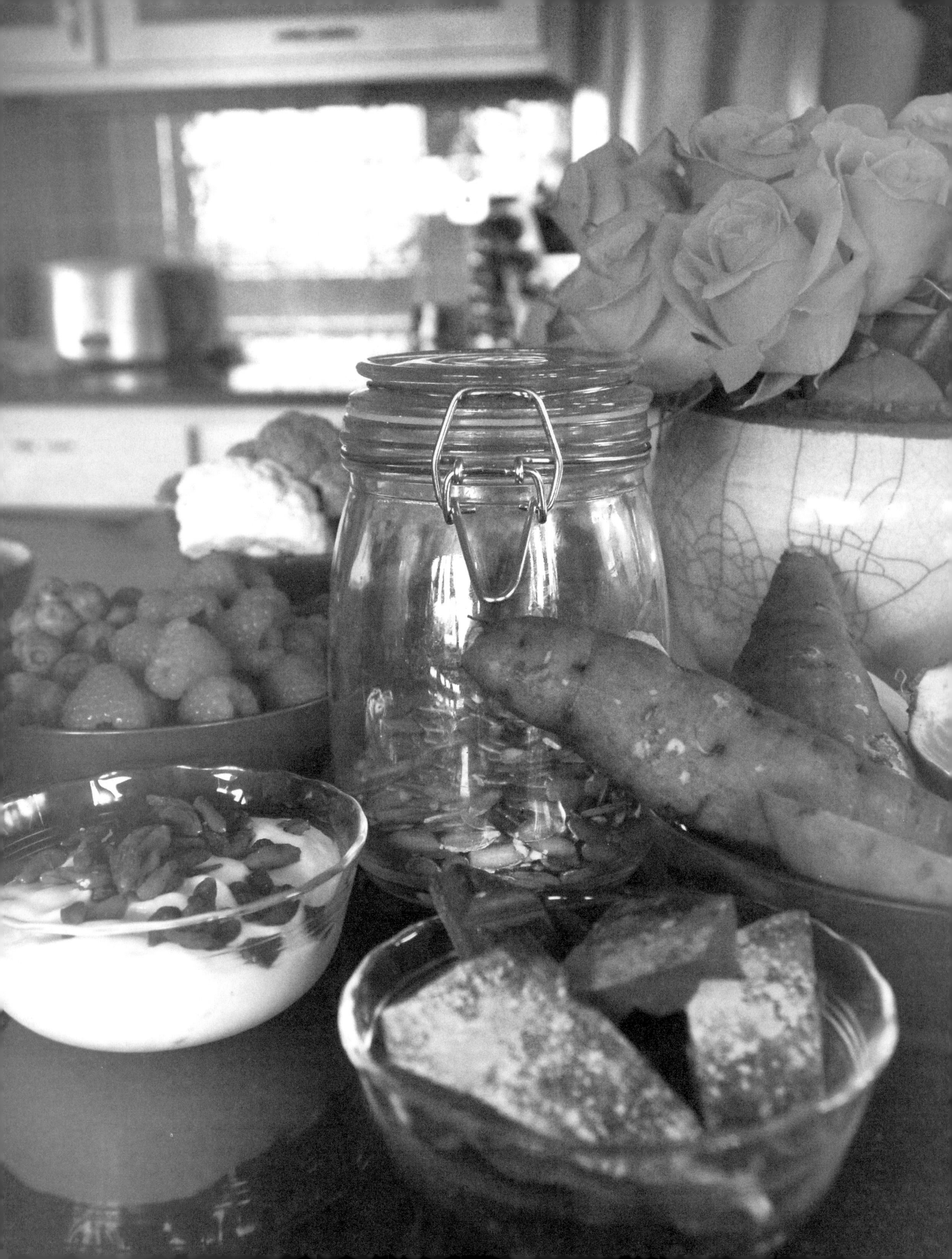

The Fertile Soul's Pantry

How do we start? The first step, and maybe the most important component, is stocking the pantry. We want you to continue to nourish your Fertile Soul by having easy access to healthful alternatives that you love! This list contains many delicious "fertility friendly" choices. Many health food stores offer lists of "wheat free," "gluten free," "low glycemic" and "dairy free" products. Use these lists on your journey to discovering brands that create healthy "fertility friendly" products.

Refined carbohydrates and wheat alternatives:

In place of wheat, look for sprouted breads (e.g., Ezekial, Food for Life) and products made with spelt flour, rice flour, oat flour, corn flour and polenta. Choose brown rice over white rice. Use pasta alternatives including spelt, brown rice, spaghetti squash and quinoa. It is important to note that having wheat sensitivity is different than being diagnosed with gluten intolerance. If you have been diagnosed with gluten intolerance or Celiac disease, please also avoid the products marked (G) below.

When shopping, it should be safe to purchase products marked gluten-free, as the manufacturer is assuring that their products will not contain wheat.

[NOTE: If you question whether you might have gluten intolerance, try eliminating (G) products for three weeks, and take note of how you feel. If you have gluten sensitivity, when you allow gluten back in the diet, it may make you may feel sick, tired, or "hung-over." If not, feel safe allowing the grain back into your diet.]

WHOLE GRAINS: have a look at cooking whole grains in "Break the fast" to learn how to prepare these delicious grains.

- Amaranth
- Barley (G)
- Buckwheat
- Flaxseed
- Kamut (G)
- Millet
- Oat (G)
- Quinoa
- Brown Rice
- Rye (G)
- Spelt (G)
- Sprouted Wheat
- Teff

FLOURS: When baking with gluten-free flours, using a small amount of tapioca flour can be helpful in creating a mixture that holds together. My husband often says gluten-free baking is for the birds that get to pick up the leftover crumbles!

- Almond
- Buckwheat
- Tapioca
- Chestnut
- Chickpea
- Coconut
- Hazelnut
- Jerusalem artichoke
- Kamut (G)
- Sorghum
- Oat (G)
- Brown Rice
- Rye (G)

PASTAS: cook wheat-free and gluten-free pastas just a little less time than refined pasta for a good "al dente" Italian experience.

- Kamut (G)
- Quinoa
- Spelt (G)
- Brown Rice

COOKING OILS: use olive oil at medium heat only; sesame oil and ghee are preferable for high heat cooking.

- Unrefined extra virgin olive
- Unrefined organic sesame
- Clarified butter/ghee (see Basic Ingredients)

TOPPING OILS AND HEALTHY FAT SOURCES: since our hormones are stored in our fat cells, using healthy oils is essential for balanced endocrine health.

- Unrefined extra virgin olive oil
- Usana Optomega
- Evening Primrose
- Black current
- Pumpkin seed
- Chia seed
- Avocado
- Nuts and seeds

COW DAIRY ALTERNATIVES: trying the alternatives below for at least one month is a great way to realize if you are sensitive to the more complex protein structure in cow dairy. Where possible avoid the aseptic Tetra Pak packaging often used by almond and hemp milks by making your own (see Hydrate). The aluminum can seep through the thin plastic coating and contaminate your milk product.

- Goat or sheep milk, yogurt and cheese
- Almond milk and cheese
- Hemp milk
- Soy milk creamer

ROOM TEMPERATURE BEVERAGES: your digestive system thrives when you avoid ice-cold beverages. Pass on ice and prefer warmer beverages.

- Hot Lemon Water
- Herbal teas
- Water
- Sparkling water (with or without a splash of unsweetened juice)
- Kombucha
- Tea Chino

ORGANIC PROTEIN SOURCES: a palm-sized portion of protein helps to stabilize blood sugar levels at each meal. Grains and greens also contain protein, so remember to use meats as a condiment and not a main course.

- Wild Salmon
- Tempeh
- Tofu
- Nuts and nut butters (see Basic Ingredients)
- Beans and legumes (on the side)
- Seeds
- Ground turkey
- Grass fed chicken
- Free-range egg yolks or egg alternative (see Basic Ingredients)
- Organic beef

VEGETABLES: Choose seasonal local and organic produce to stay in harmony with nature. Cruciferous vegetables help to metabolize excess estradiol, while dark leafy greens provide nourishing chlorophyll content.

- Broccoli
- Brussels Sprouts
- Chard

- Kale
- Cauliflower
- Yams/ sweet potatoes
- Dark leafy greens (kale, spinach, collard)
- Seaweed
- Asparagus
- Snow peas
- Zucchini
- Carrots

FRUIT: It is always best to consume fruits in their whole form rather than overly sweet fruit juices that contain a lot of sugar.

- Pear
- Apple
- Pineapple
- Mango
- Goji berries
- Raspberry
- Blueberry
- Blackberry
- Strawberry
- Lemon and lime
- Avocadoes
- Cranberries
- Oranges
- Pomegranate
- Peaches

LOW-GLYCEMIC SWEETENERS: Ideally we would avoid sweeteners as much as possible, which contribute to "dampness" and yeast overgrowth. For occasional use, experiment with some of the options below instead of refined and artificial varieties. You will likely notice your cravings for overly sweet foods will disappear as you practice the guidelines in this book.

- Agave Syrup
- Xylitol
- Erythritol
- Yacon sweetener
- Green Stevia

Basic ingredients you can make at home...

Clarified butter or ghee *is butter that has had the milk solids removed.* One advantage it has is a much higher smoke point, so you can cook with it at higher temperatures without its browning and burning. It also can be kept for much longer than regular butter without going rancid.

8 tablespoons butter = 6 tablespoons ghee

To make ghee, melt a stick of butter slowly. Let it sit for a bit; it will separate. Skim off the foam that rises to the top and gently pour the butter off, discarding the milk solids that have settled to the bottom. Store for up to six months.

Egg replacer *has the benefit of omega 3 fatty acids from the flaxseed.* If you have Liver or Gall bladder excess conditions including migraine headaches, PMS and skin irritations, use egg replacer when baking or cooking.

1 egg =

1 tablespoon ground flaxseed meal + 3 tablespoons hot water

Combine flaxseed meal and water, using a hand mixer on high for one minute. Use immediately.

Nut butters *provide a good source of protein and fat.*

2 cups organic nuts (almonds, cashews, hazelnuts, walnuts)

2 tablespoons unrefined sesame oil

Salt to taste

Soak nuts in water overnight. Combine nuts and salt in food processor, chopping until finely ground. Add oil and continue to mix until desired texture.

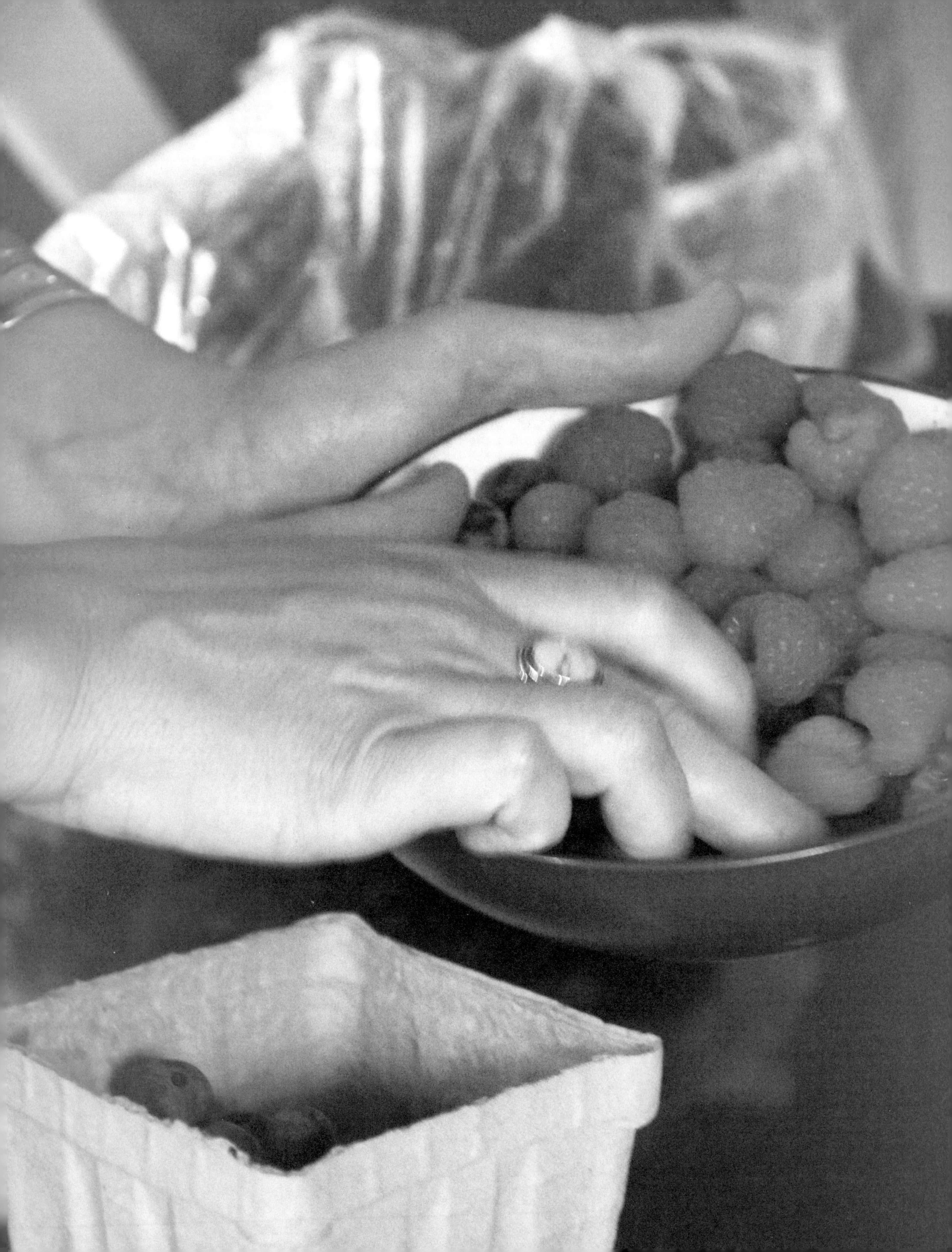

Enjoying Cooking for Fertility...

1. *At the beginning of each recipe you will find a short paragraph that details the healing benefits of the foods you will be preparing and eating.*
2. *If there is a particular food you enjoy, please look to the Glossary and Index to learn how this edible can benefit your reproductive function, as well as other dishes you might also enjoy.*
3. *If you are interested in addressing specific symptoms or aligning your eating plan with the cycles of the moon, meal plans, shopping lists and lifestyle guidelines are available in the Appendix.*
4. *If you are new to cooking or feel you might benefit from some additional support on how to prepare meals to enhance your fertility, consider purchasing the Cooking for Fertility DVD at www.cookingforfertility.com.*
5. *Most importantly, experiment with and enjoy all of the dishes in this cookbook. They have been designed to nourish you and your fertility.*

Bon Appetit!

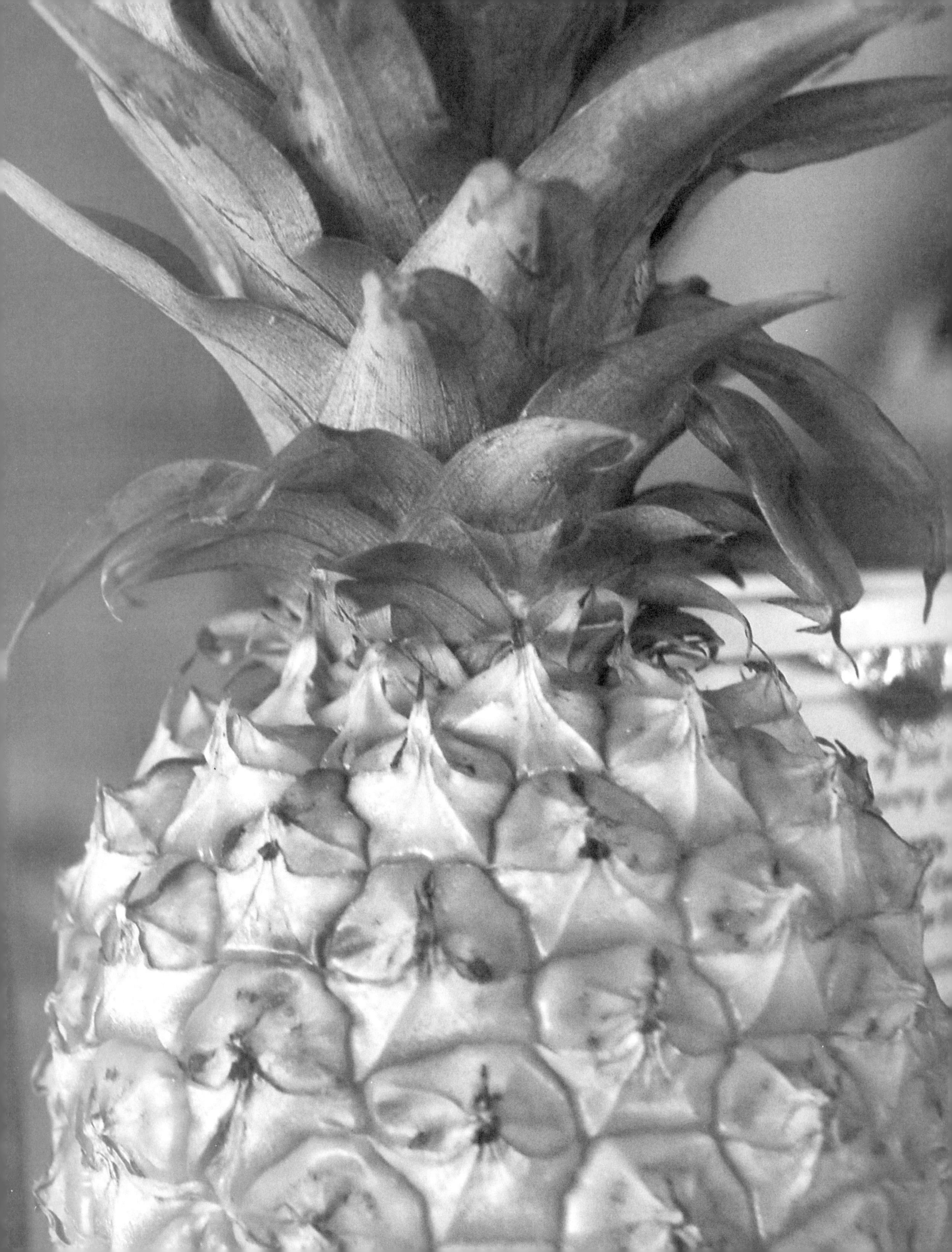

Break the fast

- The word for the first meal of the day summarizes literally what you are doing as you break your night-long fast. After restoring yourself with a full night of sleep, your body utilizes breakfast's nutrients to fuel the day's activities. Your fertility needs breakfast.
- From the Chinese medicine view, the hours from 7 to 11 a.m. correspond with the peak spleen and stomach energies, making this the perfect time to consume nourishing foods.
- A balanced protein and carbohydrate meal in the morning raises your metabolism and helps ensure stable blood sugar and energy levels throughout the day, giving your body's systems, including your reproductive organs, the fuel they need for proper function.

BREAKFAST ON THE FLY

Making a few minutes for mindful eating is important. Preparing breakfast doesn't have to take a lot of time, and doing so is well worth it.

GRAINS TO GO

Combine 1/2 cup of rolled oats or quinoa with 1 1/2 cups boiling water in a widemouthed thermos and seal tightly, leaving overnight. Add toppings such as berries, walnuts, or flaxseed in the morning, and you are on your way!

FERTILE ALTERNATIVES TO COMMON BREAKFAST CHOICES

I learned from Paul Pitchford that using whole eggs appears to directly contribute to PCOS and issues of infertility.[14] Since studying with him, I personally only use the egg yolks to avoid mucous issues created by the whites. According to the USDA the egg yolks contain much more nutritional value than the egg whites, with a concentration of essential fatty acids and vitamins.[15] Current research at the University of Surrey has shown that saturated fat in the diet from pastries, processed meats and baked goods has more adverse effects on cholesterol levels than eating cholesterol-rich foods like eggs.[16]

Instead of a fried egg, boil organic, free-range eggs for 10-12 minutes for hardboiled or 3-4 minutes for soft-boiled. Toast sprouted whole-grain bread and serve with pureed or sliced avocado instead of butter.

Replace bacon with organic turkey bacon, vegetarian bacon, chicken-apple sausage, tempeh, or beans.

Substitute morning coffee with tea chino using healing herbal teas.

Instead of the familiar peanut butter and jelly sandwich on refined white or wheat bread, try spreading walnut, almond, sunflower seed, cashew or pumpkin seed butters over sprouted breads, rice flour or spelt English muffins.

Replace morning juice with fresh whole fruits such as pineapples, mangoes, raspberries, blueberries and blackberries. Apples and pears are delicious served with goat-milk yogurt.

COOKING WHOLE GRAINS

Whole grains are a staple of the Fertility Diet, and you can enjoy them prepared in a variety of ways at every meal. Complex carbohydrates help overcome sugar cravings, support digestion, stabilize mood, boost energy levels and promote restful sleep. Grains foster a peaceful mind and induce a state of receptivity and relaxation that nurtures your most fertile state.[17]

A guide for cooking everyday grains

The table below will guide you in experimenting with different wheat-free grains. It is a good practice to rinse your grains prior to cooking to remove any debris. You may also soak the grains overnight to reduce cooking time and save energy. As a general rule, cooked grains will yield two-to-three times the amount of the dry grains you initially added.

1 Cup Dry	Water	Simmer	TCM Imbalance	Notable Nutrients	Gluten
Amaranth	3 cups	25–30 minutes	Dampness	Protein, fiber, amino acids, vitamin C calcium	No
Barley	3 cups	1½ hrs.	Heart, Kidney Yin, Spleen, Dampness, Heat	Fiber, calcium, iron, protein	Yes
Cornmeal (Polenta)	3 cups	30 minutes	Heart, Dampness	Protein, iron, manganese, potassium	No
Millet	2 cups	30 minutes	Kidney Yin, Heat	Iron, silicon	No
Rolled Oats	2 cups	30 minutes	Heart, Spleen	Silicon, phosphorus	Yes
Quinoa	2 cups	20 minutes	Kidney Yang	Protein, calcium, iron, phosphorus, B vitamins, vitamin E	No
Brown Rice	2 cups	45 minutes	Heart, Spleen, Kidney yang	Vitamin E, polysaccharides, trace minerals, Alpha lipoic acid, CoQ10	No
Spelt Flakes	3 cups	25–30 minutes	Spleen and Kidney Yang	Protein, fiber, manganese, B3, magnesium	Yes

GOURMET OATMEAL

Oats add substance to the diet, calming the nervous system and inviting the relaxation response so important to fertility. Walnuts and flaxseed are full of omega-3 fatty acids, and adding dark berries provides antioxidants to nourish blood and support its flow. Oatmeal is a very nutritious breakfast. Slowly simmered in water, oatmeal benefits the reproductive organs and sets the stage for stable blood sugar and energy levels all day.

Serves 2
Cooking time: 20-30 minutes

3 cups water

1 1/2 cups rolled oats

1/4 cup raisins

1/2 cup blueberries

2 teaspoons ground flaxseed

1/4 cup crushed walnuts

2 tablespoons applesauce (optional)

Bring water to a boil. Add oats and simmer on medium heat. Once the water evaporates, add raisins and berries. Place in a bowl and top with flaxseed, walnuts, and/or applesauce, if desired.

APPLESAUCE

The reproductive organs, which correspond to the Water element in TCM, respond to foods simmered slowly in liquid. Apples are cooling in nature and nourish your yin, which is often depleted by stress and our fast-paced lifestyles. Apples benefit people with low blood sugar or emotional depression.[18] Cinnamon invigorates the digestive fire and combines with the low-glycemic sweetener, agave nectar, to delight the palate. Enjoy a dollop of applesauce on top of your morning grains.

Serves 4
Cooking time: 12 minutes

4 medium apples, cored, quartered and peeled

1/2 cup water

1 stick of cinnamon (or 1/2 tsp ground)

1/4 cup agave nectar (optional)

Combine apples, water and cinnamon stick in a saucepan. Cover and simmer for 10 minutes or until apples are tender. Remove cinnamon stick and mash apples. Stir in agave nectar, if desired, and serve.

QUINOA, THE MOTHER OF GRAINS

Quinoa packs 16% more protein than any other grain, warming you from the inside out. Its plant protein contains manganese, magnesium, iron, and all nine essential amino acids.[19] Soaking quinoa overnight helps to release nutrients and improves digestibility. Nurture yourself with this nutrient-dense start to the day or enjoy with lunch or dinner as a savory side dish.

Serves 2
Cooking time: 35 minutes

2 cups water

1 cup quinoa, soaked

1/2 cup steamed almond, hemp or goat milk

1/4 cup slivered almonds

1/2 cup raspberries

1/4 tsp cinnamon

1 teaspoon flaxseed

Place water and quinoa in a covered saucepan. Bring to a boil, reduce heat to low and simmer for 30 minutes. Turn off heat and let sit 5 minutes. Uncover and add almonds, raspberries, steamed milk and cinnamon.

ROOT CONGEE

Congees are Asian porridges. The simplest congees consist of rice simmered slowly in abundant amounts of water. Often other grains and ingredients are added for flavor and nutrients. This cooking method is beneficial to both reproductive and digestive function.[20] Root vegetables have a grounding quality that provides wonderful sustenance for the day ahead.

Yields 3-4 cups
Cooking time: 3-4 hours

1 cup grain (brown rice, oats, amaranth, millet, barley or quinoa)

7 cups water (add less if you desire a thicker congee)

1/2 cup sweet potatoes, cooked and cubed

1/2 teaspoon cinnamon

1/4 teaspoon nutmeg

1/4 cup goji berries

1/2 cup crushed nuts to top

In a large pot, bring water and grain to a boil. Add in cubed root vegetables with nutmeg, cinnamon and goji berries. Reduce to low heat and simmer for 3-4 hours. Top with nuts and serve.

GRANOLA

Oats contain complex carbohydrates and nutrients that help regulate cellular health including immune response and neurotransmitter function.[21] This recipe is packed with many fertility-enhancing additions: goji berries to nourish the blood, almonds to provide vitamin E, walnuts and pumpkin seeds for omegas and zinc, and low glycemic index agave nectar, to add a touch of sweetness. Enjoy on top of goat milk yogurt or with almond milk (see Hydrate).

Yields 7-8 cups
Cooking time: 45 minutes, 300 degrees

4 cups large rolled oats
1/4 cup almonds, chopped
1/4 cup walnuts, chopped
1/4 cup unsweetened coconut
1 teaspoon cinnamon
1/4 cup pumpkin seeds
1/4 cup agave syrup
1 teaspoon vanilla
1/2 cup sesame seed butter
1/4 cup water
1 tsp flaxseed
1 cup dried fruits (any combination of goji berries, cranberries, apricots, dates, raisins, blueberries)

Preheat oven to 300 degrees. Lightly grease baking pan with clarified butter or olive oil cooking spray. In a large bowl, combine oats, nuts, coconut, cinnamon and seeds. In a separate bowl, mix agave syrup, vanilla, sesame butter and water, and blend thoroughly. Stir into dry mixture and pour onto pan. Bake for 45 minutes, or until golden brown, stirring every 15 minutes to avoid burning the sides. Remove from heat, cool, add dried fruit and flaxseed and mix well.

SPROUTED FERTILITY LOAF

Featured recipe in Cooking for Fertility DVD with Tiffany Pollard and Kathryn Flynn

Sprouted grains help to reduce inflammation, counteracting the impact of wheat and refined carbohydrates. Sprouts are high in nutrients and help create an optimal environment for conception and implantation. The addition of sprouted pumpkin seeds provides a dose of healthful omega-3 fatty acids and zinc. Red clover contains vitamin B, thiamine, vitamin C, and calcium, which help relax the nervous system and alkalize cervical mucous, creating an ideal PH balance in the uterus.[22] Top with delicious nut butter for a balanced protein-carbohydrate start to the day.

Yields 1 medium loaf
Cooking time: 1 hour, 350 degrees

Sprouting instructions: In two separate bowls, jars or pots soak quinoa and pumpkin seeds overnight; use enough water to cover the grains and seeds by 3 to 4 inches. The next morning drain, rinse with cool water and drain again. Repeat this procedure twice a day, for one to two days until you see sprouts of approximately 1/4 inch.

2 cups quinoa seeds

1/2 cup pumpkin seeds

1/4 cup red clover

1 teaspoon cinnamon

1/4 cup apple juice

3 tablespoon agave nectar

2 to 3 tablespoons unrefined olive oil for drizzling on top

Preheat oven to 350 degrees. Combine sprouted seeds, red clover, cinnamon, agave and apple juice in a large bowl. Transfer mixture to a food processor and blend until smooth "dough like" consistency is achieved. Place loaf mixture in a lightly greased loaf pan and bake for approximately 1 hour or more until golden brown on top and cooked through. Try drizzling some unrefined olive oil on top just after it comes out of the oven.

YAM SCONES

If you can find the African variety of yams, which are white, they could increase your odds of having twins![23] Enjoy these delicious sweet scones topped with omega-rich walnuts. Avoid in cases of Polycystic Ovarian Syndrome (PCOS).

Yields 4-6 large scones
Cooking time: 30-45 minutes, 375 degrees

1 cup cooked yams, mashed

2 egg yolks or egg substitute (see basic ingredients)

2 tablespoons agave nectar

2 tablespoons olive oil

1 teaspoon vanilla

1 cup brown rice or almond flour

1 cup tapioca flour

1/4 teaspoon xanthum gum

1/2 teaspoon Chinese allspice

1 1/2 tablespoons fresh ginger

1 tablespoon crushed walnuts

Beat together yams, eggs, agave, olive oil, and vanilla. In a separate bowl, combine all dry ingredients. Slowly fold wet ingredients into dry mixture until mixture is thick. Add dollops of your desired size on a greased baking sheet and top with walnut pieces. Bake at 375 degrees for 30-45 minutes until golden brown. Best served immediately with ghee (see Basic Ingredients).

GOJI NUT MUFFINS

Nuts are a great source of protein and fat. Almonds and pumpkin seeds add omegas, vitamin E and zinc. Goji berries nourish the blood, which feeds the ovaries and uterus. In the summer, experiment with adding seasonal blueberries, raspberries or blackberries for even more antioxidants.

Yields 9-12 muffins
Cooking time: 15-20 minutes, 375 degrees

2 cups almonds

1/2 cup pumpkin seeds

2 egg yolks or egg substitute (see Basic Ingredients)

1/4 cup melted clarified butter

1/3 cup agave syrup

1 teaspoon vanilla

1/2 teaspoon baking soda

1/2 cup goji berries

1/2 cup seasonal blueberries, raspberries and blackberries (optional)

In a food processor, grind almonds and pumpkin seeds until smooth. Beat in eggs. Add clarified butter, agave nectar and vanilla. Mix fully, then fold in goji berries and baking soda. Spoon the mixture into muffin tins lined with paper cups. Bake at 375 degrees for 15-20 minutes. Muffins will have a golden brown top but will not rise.

EGG BURRITO

Eggs nourish and build the blood to support reproductive function. They are an excellent source of protein and vitamin B12. If you have premenstrual symptoms including irritability, headaches, or breast tenderness at ovulation, omit egg whites and use only the yolk (unless you have problems with cholesterol), or opt for tofu scramble (recipe later in this section).

Serves 2
Cooking time: 10-12 minutes

2 sprouted-grain spelt tortillas or 4 corn tortillas

4 egg yolks

1/4 cup almond, hemp or goat milk

1 teaspoon extra virgin olive oil

1 medium-sized avocado, sliced

Salsa to taste

2 tablespoons goat cheese

Warm tortillas over low heat in a skillet or use toaster oven. Whisk together eggs and milk alternative; pour into saucepan and scramble over medium heat with olive oil. Place 1/4 of egg mixture in each tortilla and top with avocado, salsa and crumbled goat cheese if desired.

THE CONSCIOUS FRITTATA

How we eat may be more important than What we eat!

There is a culinary chicken-and-the-egg situation at play. The foods (What) we eat affect our body and How we eat, feel/think also creates an environment of bio-chemicals, hormones and endorphins inside our body which in turn affects how our foods process. Start your day off with ease and grace. Eggs are a great source of choline, which is essential for brain health. And eggs, of course, are an age-old symbol of fertility!

Serves 2
Cooking time: 15-20 minutes

1 tsp extra virgin olive oil

4 organic, free-range eggs

2 tablespoons sliced black olives

1 tablespoon julienne sliced sun-dried tomatoes

1 celery stalk/rib thinly sliced

2 basil leaves sliced into thin strips

4 sliced crimini mushrooms

1/3 cup grated cheese (optional)

a dash of cumin, cinnamon, salt and pepper

Beat the eggs in a bowl while slightly browning the mushrooms in a pan with olive oil. Add the other ingredients to your eggs and beat again. Pour the egg mixture into the pan and let cook for a while until the bottom starts to feel solid (gently jiggle the pan). If you chose to add the grated cheese, do that now and then instead of flipping (and tearing) the frittata, put the pan underneath your broiler and keep watch until the top is golden brown.Serve on a slice of toasted sprouted or rye bread with your favorite. Eat without distractions and with a smile.

This recipe is by *EatWell, LiveWell, LoveWell, Culinary Consciousness Coach Caspar Poyck C.Ht.*

www.consciouslyliving.com

ROOT HASH TRIO

Root hash is a perfect way to clean out the fridge at the end of the week and enjoy a leisurely weekend brunch that's not the usual breakfast fare. The combination of leafy greens, root vegetables and mushrooms strengthens the entire body and helps build immunity. Polenta, which is ground corn, is a heart nourishing grain that promotes vitality in the sexual organs.[24] If you want to save time in the morning, make the polenta the night before.

Serves 2
Cooking time: 60 minutes, 375 degrees

1 cup polenta

3 cups water

1/2 cup root vegetables, sliced (winter squash, rutabaga, parsnip, carrot, turnip)

1/2 cup leafy greens, chopped (kale, collards, red chard)

1/4 cup mushrooms, halved (shiitake, button, crimini)

4 tablespoons extra virgin olive oil (save 1/2 tablespoon for polenta)

Sea salt or dulse flakes to taste

4 egg yolks

Bring water to a boil in a medium pot. Add polenta and let simmer for 30 minutes. Remove from heat, pour into cake pan and let cool. Preheat oven to 375 degrees. Place root vegetables, greens and mushrooms in a 9 x 9 glass pan. Roast in oven for approximately 40 minutes. Drizzle with olive oil and flavor with salt or dulse flakes as desired. While vegetables are roasting, fill saucepan with water to about two-thirds and bring to a boil. Add eggs, reduce heat to medium, and simmer for approximately 10 minutes. In a separate skillet, heat 1/2 tablespoon olive oil. Cut two portions of polenta the size of a slice of bread and lightly pan-fry them on medium heat. Layer food on plate, starting with polenta, followed by roasted root vegetables, and topped with egg.

OMEGA-3 BENEDICT OVER SPINACH

Free-range eggs and salmon contain a healthy dose of omega-3 fatty acids. Spinach fills us with iron and chlorophyll, which helps to build blood. This dish is particularly beneficial in cases of scanty blood flow, short cycles and amenorrhea. Use last night's wild salmon (a great fish to eat at least 2-3 times a week) and cover with the delicious almost-hollandaise sauce!

Serves 2
Cooking time: 45-60 minutes

4 free-range eggs, poached

2 cups spinach

1 cooked salmon fillet

2 medium avocados, sliced

1/2 tablespoon olive oil

3/4 cup almost-hollandaise sauce

Fill saucepan two-thirds full with water and bring to a boil. Add eggs, reduce heat to medium and simmer for approximately 10 minutes. Steam spinach in a colander until bright green. In a separate skillet, heat olive oil. Lightly pan-fry salmon on medium heat until warm. Layer spinach, salmon, eggs, avocado and the almost-hollandaise sauce below.

Almost hollandaise sauce

Yields: 1/2 cup
Cooking time: 15-20 minutes

2 egg yolks

1/2 cup goat yogurt

1 1/2 teaspoons lemon juice

1/4 tsp Dijon mustard

1/2 tablespoon dill (fresh or dried)

In a saucepan, whisk together eggs, yogurt and lemon juice at low heat. Stir consistently for 15-20 minutes, until desired thickness is attained. Remove from heat and stir in mustard and dill.

TOFU SCRAMBLE

Tofu cools an overly stressed-out reproductive system by reducing heat accumulated as a result of a busy lifestyle, overwork, poor diet and other unhealthy habits. Mushrooms build immunity, and turmeric helps to reduce inflammation, a precursor to many chronic diseases, and increases blood flow to the uterus and ovaries.

Serves 2
Cooking time: 10-15 minutes

1 teaspoon extra virgin olive oil
1/4 cup red onion, chopped
1 tablespoon red bell pepper, diced
1/2 cup shiitake mushrooms, diced
1 1/2 cups firm tofu, crumbled
1 teaspoon dried thyme
1 teaspoon rosemary
2 garlic cloves, crushed
1/2 teaspoon turmeric
Sea salt to taste

In a skillet, sauté olive oil and vegetables until softened. Add tofu and seasoning, cooking until liquid evaporates.

PINEAPPLE FRENCH TOAST

Why do we crave sweets? Chinese Medicine teaches that the sweet flavor enters the Spleen and can help balance mild cases of Liver Stagnation, which can cause PMS. As an additional bonus, pineapple contains bromelain, an enzyme helpful in promoting implantation. In cases of Dampness, candida (systemic yeast) or excess weight, eliminate syrups and avoid all sweet foods.

Serves 2
Cooking time: 10 minutes

2 egg yolks

1/4 cup almond milk

1 teaspoon cinnamon

4 pieces spelt bread

1 tablespoon extra virgin olive oil

2 tablespoons pineapple syrup

1/2 cup fresh pineapple cubes (optional)

In a large bowl, combine eggs, almond milk and cinnamon. Lightly baste bread with egg mixture and place in heated frying pan with olive oil. Cook at medium heat, flipping once. Top with pineapple syrup and fresh pineapple.

Pineapple syrup

Yields: 1 cup
Cooking time: 5 minutes

1/2 cup agave nectar

1/4 cup macadamia nut oil

1/2 cup fresh or frozen pineapple

Combine all ingredients in a blender, and pulse until liquefied. Heat briefly in a skillet over medium heat and drizzle over french toast.

COCO-BERRY PANCAKES

Spelt is a glutinous wheat alternative. Use egg replacer (see basic recipes) in cases of Liver Excess. Adding a handful of flaxseed benefits digestion and provides omega-3s. Raspberries regulate the menstrual cycle and manage excess bleeding, and blueberries nourish Kidney Yin, supporting the resolution of "urinary, sexual and reproductive imbalances."[25]

Serves 2-4
Cooking time: 10-15 minutes

2 cups spelt flour

1 teaspoon baking powder

1 1/2 cups coconut milk

1 tablespoon olive oil

2 eggs lightly beaten

1/4 cup agave syrup

1/4 cup blueberries or raspberries

1 tablespoon extra virgin olive oil

1 tablespoon ground flaxseed

Combine dry ingredients. In a separate bowl, mix together wet ingredients. Add wet mixture to dry mixture. Add in berries. Grease the pan with olive oil and warm over medium-low heat. Add 1/4 cup of the batter to heated saucepan and cook until bubbles form on top. Flip, and cook 2-3 minutes more until done. Serve drizzled with simple syrup.

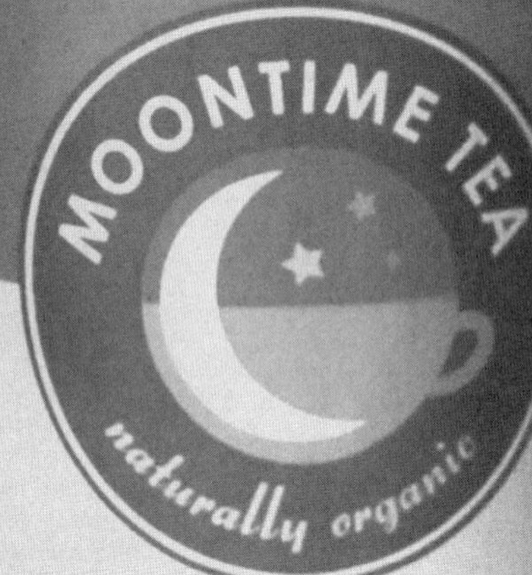
MOONTIME TEA
naturally organic

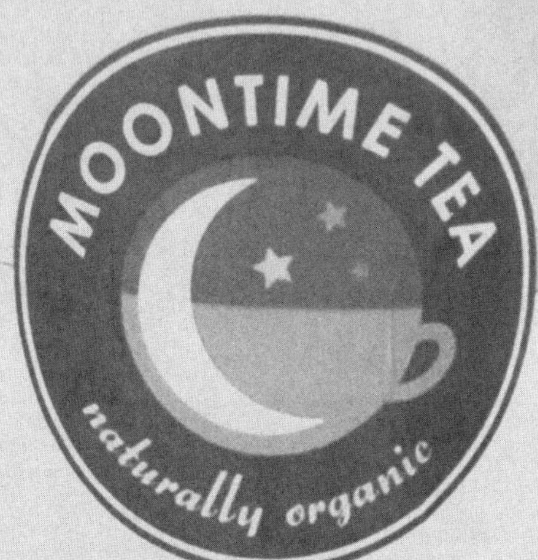
MOONTIME TEA
naturally organic

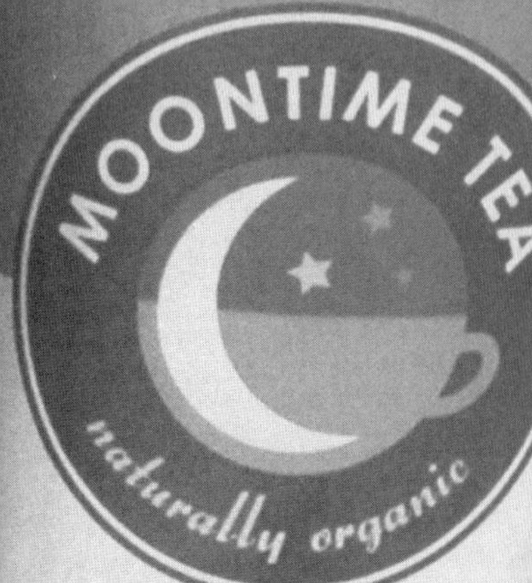
MOONTIME TEA
naturally organic

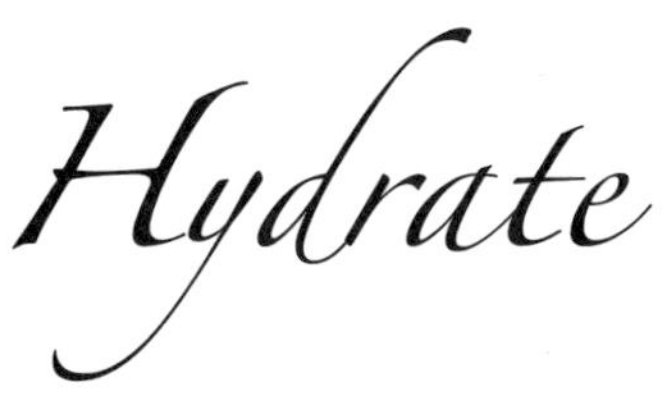

- First thing in the morning, drink a cup of hot water with fresh-squeezed lemon to help detoxify the liver and aid digestion.
- Keep hydrated by drinking water and herbal tea throughout the day. Listen to your body's wisdom to guide you on how much liquid to consume.
- Drink room-temperature beverages before and after meals, not during. Cold drinks like ice water and frozen beverages can put out your digestive fire, forcing the Spleen to work harder to reheat and break down nutrients.
- Juice fasts are common in intense detoxification programs. Yet, with fertility, you want to replenish your system and use gentle methods of detoxification like sea-salt foot soaks and lavender baths. The summer is the best time to drink fresh juices; adding fresh ginger keeps digestive fire strong.
- Kombucha or homemade soda (recipes to follow) are good replacements for commercial sodas, most of which are loaded with caffeine and sugar or artificial sweeteners. Recent studies have shown that caffeine increases the risk of miscarriage. High sugar content is also undesirable for fertility, and ingredients such as Aspartame raise prolactin levels, which interferes with ovulation. Carbonated beverages can also leach calcium (needed for fetal bone growth) from your bones.
- Replace coffee, both caffeinated and decaffeinated, with herbal teas. Not only can caffeine increase the chance of miscarriage, it also drains the adrenals and saps reproductive energies. Need a Starbucks fix? Ask for a tea misto with steamed soymilk.

FRESH HERBAL TEA INFUSIONS WITH HEALING PROPERTIES

Chamomile is calming and gently detoxifies the liver, relieving headaches, anxiety and menstrual cramps.

Peppermint helps cool an overstressed system and relieve symptoms of PMS and other stagnations in the body.

Nettles are full of nutrients, and help increase energy and nourish the blood.

Ginger supports digestion and can stimulate menses.

Milk thistle soothes an overworked liver, especially during the menstrual cycle.

Red raspberry leaves are believed to tone the uterus, support conception and prevent pregnancy complications.

Red clover enhances fertility and helps regulate menstrual cycles. Because of its blood-thinning qualities, it is not recommended for women with heavy bleeding.

BREWING TEA

To prepare hot tea, add 1 tablespoon of herbs and 1 1/2 cups boiling water to a glass container. Steep for 10 minutes. Strain liquid; remove herbs and serve. Add steamed milk alternative (see recipes for almond milk, hemp milk, and coconut milk later in this section), if desired. To prepare cold tea, follow the same procedure with cold water. Let steep for at least one hour. Serve at room temperature.

CATHY'S CHAI TEA

Chai is a staple tea in India, and often used to support digestion. If you feel cold most of the time or have cold feet and hands (which can also mean a Cold Uterus), drink chai while soaking your feet in warm water and Epsom salts. Cardamom, cinnamon, cloves, and pepper are wonderfully warming spices to include in tea. They help invigorate blood flow and move stagnant energy, alleviating conditions of fibroids, endometriosis and PMS.

Yields: 5-6 cups

7 cups water (a full medium pot)

8 cardamom pods, crushed

10 cloves, crushed

3/4 teaspoon black peppercorns, crushed

1 tablespoon cinnamon or 1 cinnamon stick

1/4 inch piece fresh ginger, finely grated

2 bags decaffeinated black or redbush tea

Optional: almond, goat, or hemp milk

Add cardamom, cloves, pepper, cinnamon and ginger to water and bring to a boil. Reduce to medium-low. Add decaf black tea, steeping for 3 minutes, or use redbush tea and leave in. Simmer on medium for 20 minutes. Add steamed or cold milk alternative, if desired.

TEA CHINO

Tea preferentially dilates blood vessels in the body and does not contain any of the harmful oils present in both caffeinated and decaffeinated coffee. This drink is often called Tea Misto at popular coffee chains. It offers a healthful alternative to the traditional latte.

Yields: 3-4 cups

4 cups water

2 bags herbal tea (tea chino recommended)

1 cup steamed, almond, hemp or goat milk

Optional: simple syrup or agave nectar to taste

Bring water to a boil, remove it from the heat and add the tea chino. Steep about 10 minutes, until the whole pot is flavored. While the tea is steeping, steam the milk alternative. Pour tea, add the foamed milk and sweeten if desired.

KOMBUCHA

In China, kombucha has been referred to as the "Elixir of Life." This fermented beverage contains many beneficial probiotics, enzymes, vitamins and amino acids. Drinking kombucha helps restore healthy flora balance to the gut and contributes to improved digestion, immunity, metabolism, cellular development and liver function. This is not a sweet tea, as the sugar is utilized in the fermentation process. The drink itself tastes somewhat acidic, but it makes the body and cervical mucus more alkaline, creating an ideal environment for implantation.

Yields: 5-6 cups

7 cups purified water

1 kombucha starter (scoby)

4-6 bags black decaffeinated tea

1 cup organic sugar

In a large pot, bring water to a boil, add tea bags, and turn off heat. Soak for approximately 15 minutes. Remove tea bags, add sugar, and let mixture cool. Add kombucha starter into a clean 3 liter bowl and cover with cheese cloth, then place in a dark, sterile area and leave undisturbed for up to three weeks. During this time the starter or scoby will multiply and you will have a "mother" to consume now and a "baby" kombucha starter for your next batch. After the waiting period set aside the starter, as you will utilize them for later batches. Place the "mother" kombucha in jars and refrigerate.

HOTTA CHOCOLATTA

Dark chocolate, a friendly monounsaturated fat, has some strong benefits for fertility. Research shows that the smell of chocolate can increase the brain's theta waves, which promote the relaxation response. Chocolate contains flavanoids known to help elevate mood, promote blood flow, ease inflammation and inhibit the formation of blood clots.[26] Chocolate also contains arginine, which increases blood flow to the uterus and ovaries specifically. Both chocolate and L-arginine supplements are best avoided in cases of Heat, and particularly if you have skin eruptions like herpes. Drink Hotta Chocolatta as an occasional treat, not an everyday staple.

Yields: 2 generous servings

2 cups almond, hemp or goat milk

1/3 cup water

2 tablespoons dark cocoa powder

1/4 teaspoon vanilla

1/4 teaspoon cinnamon

1 tablespoon agave nectar

Heat milk and water over medium-low heat. Add in cocoa powder, stirring vigorously until completely dissolved. Add remaining ingredients and stir for two minutes. Once it is simmering, remove from heat and serve while hot.

ALMOND MILK

The calcium in cow's milk is bound to the protein cassein, which is difficult for the body to break down. Almonds are an excellent source of protein, and contain zinc and vitamin E, which support the health of the uterine lining and the placenta during pregnancy. In ancient cultures, both the pagans and Romans used almonds as symbols of fertility. Enjoy almond milk frothed in tea, poured over oatmeal or blended in your berry smoothie.

Yields: 2 1/2 to 3 cups

1 cup almonds, pre-soaked overnight

3 cups water

1 tablespoon agave nectar (optional)

1 teaspoon vanilla (optional)

Blend pre-soaked almonds with water. Strain to remove pulp and put back into the blender. Add sweeteners if desired.

HEMP MILK

Hemp milk is another delightful cow dairy alternative. Hemp seeds are rich in protein, high in polyunsaturated fat and contain the perfect balance of essential fatty acids: alpha linolenic acid (omega 3) and linoleic acid (omega 6).

Yields: 2 1/2 to 3 cups

1 cup hemp seeds

3 cups purified water

In a blender mix hemp seeds with water until you see a milk-like consistency. Strain to remove pulp and put back into the blender.

COCONUT MILK

Coconut milk has a very distinctive and delicious flavor. It supports digestive function, strengthening the reproductive organs and the liver's ability to process hormones. It increases semen as well as Yin fluids, including cervical mucus. Enjoy coconut milk in our piña colada recipe and in Thai dishes and soups.

Yields: 1 1/2 to 2 cups

2 cups coconut flakes

2 cups water

Blend coconut and water. Strain and retain liquid. Use immediately or store in the refrigerator for up to one week.

PIÑA COLADA

Featured recipe in Cooking for Fertility DVD with Tiffany Pollard and Kathryn Flynn

Pineapple is particularly desirable for fertility as it contains bromelain, an enzyme known to support implantation. If you dislike pineapple, you can achieve the same results by taking digestive enzymes between meals.

Serves 2-4

1 cup fresh coconut milk

4 1/2 cups fresh or frozen pineapple

Combine pineapple in a blender with coconut milk.

MANGO LASSI

This reproductive cocktail regenerates the adrenals, kidneys and reproductive organs, which are easily taxed by our busy schedules and fast-paced lifestyles. Royal jelly strengthens reproductive function in both men and women. This is a delicious way to get a serving of full-fat dairy, which a recent Harvard medical study showed boosts fertility rates.[3]

Serves 2

1 peeled, chopped mango

2 cups goat yogurt

1/4 tsp royal jelly

Puree all ingredients in a blender until smooth.

LEMONADE AND LIMEADE

These refreshing beverages cleanse the liver and provide a high dose of vitamin C. Vitamin C improves sperm quality and supports the ovulation process. Drink a cup of hot water with lemon first thing in the morning to clear the palate and aid digestion.

Serves 2

2 cups water

1/4 cup fresh squeezed lemon or lime

1 tablespoon agave nectar

Add fresh squeezed juice of lemons or limes to water. Sweeten with agave nectar. Serve with fresh lemon or lime slices.

ALMOST SODA

Instead of drinking soda, substitute the following combination of juice and sparkling water for a fizzy satisfaction. By doing so, you will avoid harmful chemicals that disrupt the proper release and regulation of hormones and benefit from the natural nourishment of fruits and water.

Serves 2

1/2 cup limeade, lemonade or any unsweetened juice

1/2 cup sparkling water

Combine ingredients in a tall glass and enjoy!

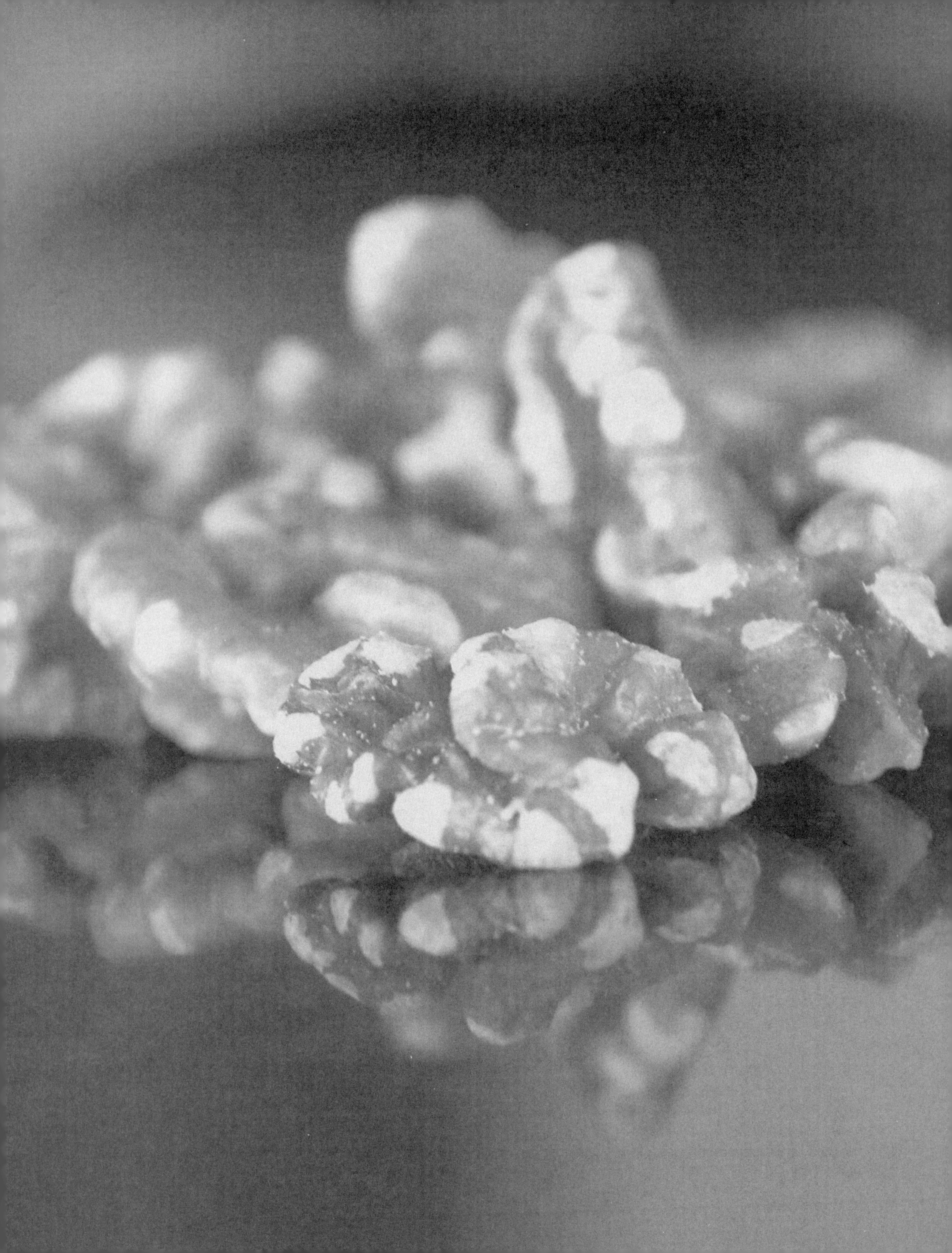

Snack and Appetize

- To boost metabolism and stabilize blood sugar levels, combine a balanced protein and carbohydrate at each meal and snack.
- Eating every three hours will help refill your energy reservoirs, curb your sugar cravings and improve your mood. Most importantly, you will reduce stress and curb fluctuations of cortisol, which impact your body's ability to conceive.
- To keep fueled throughout the day always carry some healthy snacks. Look for wheat-, sugar- and dairy-free alternatives at your local grocery store. Upon request, many stores will even provide a list of compliant product choices.
- Some of our favorite snacks-on-the-go are pumpkin seeds and goji berries, fruit and nuts, trail mix, veggie snacks, hummus and brown rice crackers, blue corn tortilla chips and guacamole, goat cheese with wheat or gluten free crackers, nut butter on sprouted toast (see Break the Fast section) and lettuce wraps (recipe follows in this section).

FRUITS AND NUTS

Fruits alkalize and cleanse the body, adding beneficial nutrients, minerals, enzymes and fiber to the diet. People who have problems with excess yeast growth (Dampness) should avoid most fruits that mold easily because of their high sugar content. For Damp conditions, pears and apples are good choices because they are less sweet. Nuts and seeds are healthful protein-rich snacks. They contain abundant essential fatty acids and vitamin E, a nerve protector, and immune-enhancing antioxidants. Nuts and seeds can increase vitality in the frail or weak; do not consume excessive nuts if you are experiencing Excess Heat or Liver Stagnation. Soak nuts in water overnight to break down their cell wall and make them easier to digest. The following table illustrates how fruits and nuts can help resolve hormonal imbalances.

TCM Condition & Healing Intention	Beneficial Fruits	Nuts and Seeds
Kidney Yang Deficiency - To generate warmth and help alleviate pre-menstrual lower back pain, frequent urination, profuse vaginal discharge	Peach, raspberry, cherry, date	Chestnut, pine nut, walnut
Kidney Yin Deficiency - To lengthen short cycles, increase cervical mucus and alleviate night sweats, hot flashes, back or knee weakness	Apple, mango, banana, blueberry, blackberry, grape, melon, mulberry, pineapple, pomegranate, raspberry, watermelon	Black sesame seed, pistachio
Liver Qi Stagnation – To alleviate premenstrual symptoms, irritability, headaches, and breast tenderness at ovulation	Peach, strawberry, orange and tangerine peel	Chestnut
Excess Heat - To reduce fevers, night sweats, hot flashes, hot skin rashes (including acne) and irritation	Apple, banana, pear, citrus, cantaloupe, persimmon, watermelon	Chia seed
Blood Stasis - To normalize blood flow and alleviate dark, brown or black menstrual blood, clotting during the period, fibroids, or endometriosis	Peach, pear, lemon, lime	All varieties nuts and seeds
Blood Deficiency - To increase scant menstrual blood and resolve premenstrual dizziness, hair loss, and dry skin	Raspberry, apricot, dried goji berries	All varieties nuts and seeds
Spleen Qi Deficiency - To improve the quality of energy in the body and reduce pre-menstrual spotting and digestive disturbances	Coconut, date	Almond, black sesame seed, flax seed, peanut, pistachio, sunflower seed
Dampness - To regulate abnormal menstrual discharges, vaginal itching and pustular skin eruptions	Cranberry, apple, pear, grapefruit, lemon peel Note: Avoid bananas	Flax seeds, chia seed, pumpkin seeds, unsalted pistachios

BERRY SMOOTHIE

Berry smoothies are delicious and healthy snacks, packed with blood-nourishing antioxidants from dark berries and balanced protein. The combination of protein and carbohydrates is essential for stabilizing blood sugar, which is particularly important in conditions of Polycystic Ovarian Syndrome (PCOS), weight loss, and for managing stress levels. When making a smoothie, thaw frozen fruit (discard juice) or combine with warm milk to balance temperature and ease digestion. Raspberries help regulate the menstrual cycle and manage excess bleeding, while blackberries have blood-building properties. Blueberries are the most cooling of the three.

Makes 2 generous servings

1 cup blueberries, raspberries, blackberries or combination

1 banana

2 cups almond, hemp or goat milk

1 tablespoon flaxseed

1-2 tablespoons whey, rice or egg protein powder

In a blender, combine all ingredients and mix at low speed until blended. Pour into glasses and serve.

GREEN SMOOTHIE

Apples, limes, avocado and mint all support the liver and replenish an overtaxed system. In Chinese Medicine, the color green corresponds to the Liver. Avocados are an excellent source of monounsaturated fat and protein and help to nourish the blood, while apples stabilize blood sugar levels and address depressive tendencies. To further cleanse the liver, mix these ingredients with wheat grass, a cereal grass high in protein, B vitamins and anti-inflammatory properties that also promotes cell regeneration.

Yields: 2 generous servings

2 green apples, unpeeled
1 ripe avocado, peeled with pit removed
1 cup unsweetened apple juice
3 sprigs mint leaves
1 tablespoon powdered wheat grass
1 teaspoon freshly squeezed lime juice
(optional: 1 oz. fresh or frozen wheat grass)

Remove the core from the apples, leaving the skin on. Pit avocado. Combine all ingredients in a blender and puree until smooth.

DOLMAS

Brown rice, pistachios and goji berries all contribute to a calm and peaceful Heart, nourishing both blood and inner spirit. In Chinese medicine, the Heart is the emperor and its only job is to pump blood. When the heart is in a state of anxiety and you feel scattered, it is important to eat Heart-nourishing foods and practice awareness in order to shift into a receptive state. Calming your nerves can be as simple as shifting your attention to the breath and being present in the moment.

Yields: 8 dolmas
Cooking time: 40-45 minutes, 375 degrees

8 grape leaves

2 cups boiling water

1 onion, chopped

1-2 tablespoons lemon juice

1 cup warm water

Stuffing:

2 teaspoons olive oil

1 cup cooked brown rice (see Cooking Grains)

1/4 cup pistachios

1/4 cup goji berries

2 tablespoons chopped parsley

3 fresh mint leaves

1/2 teaspoon ground ginger

Pour the boiling water over grape leaves. Let stand for 15 minutes, rinse in cold water and drain. Line the bottom of a casserole dish with the sliced onion. Combine stuffing ingredients. Then fill each leaf with 1 tablespoon of the prepared stuffing. Fold ends over the stuffing and roll into firm dolmas. Press tightly to secure filling. Place dolmas into the casserole dish and pour warm water on top and lemon juice over the top. Cook for 40-45 minutes at 375 degrees. Let cool and serve on a platter with babaganoush (next recipe).

BABAGANOUSH

Eggplant, lemon, mint and garlic invigorate energy flow and help resolve stagnant conditions like fibroids, endometriosis and clotting during menstruation. Eggplant contains powerful antioxidant bioflavanoids and can help resolve conditions of excess bleeding. Because eggplant promotes clearing of the uterus, it is best avoided during pregnancy[27]

Yields: 1 1/2 cups
Cooking time: 40-50 minutes, 375 degrees

2 small eggplants

2 garlic cloves

Juice of 1/2 fresh lemon

1/4 cup black sesame tahini

1 tablespoons olive oil

1/2 tablespoon fresh mint

Preheat oven to 375 degrees and bake eggplants for approximately 40 minutes until they are soft and skin is blackened. Remove insides from the eggplants and discard skin. Place in food processor with garlic, lemon juice, black sesame tahini, olive oil and mint and mix until pureed. Serve with wheat-free crackers or vegetables.

SHRIMP COCKTAIL

Shrimp is a good source of protein that builds vitality in reproductive function. Shrimp enhances yang energy (yang supports progesterone levels essential for maintaining pregnancy). Turmeric is an anti-inflammatory spice and almonds contain healthful vitamin E.

Yields: 20-25 shrimp

Cooking time: 15-20 minutes

2 lbs large shrimp, peeled with tails removed

1 tablespoon extra virgin olive oil

Paste

1/3 cup sliced or whole almonds

1 jalapeno pepper, seeded and halved

1 bunch cilantro, stems removed

6 green onions, sliced

3 cloves garlic

1 teaspoon cumin

1 teaspoon turmeric

2 tablespoons lemon juice

1 tablespoon extra virgin olive oil

Combine almonds, jalapeno pepper, cilantro, green onions, garlic, cumin, turmeric, 1 tablespoon olive oil, and lemon juice in a food processor. Blend until it forms a smooth paste. Brush shrimp with the paste and marinate in the refrigerator for at least an hour. Lightly sauté shrimp in olive oil until pink and opaque. Serve on a platter with pumpkin pesto (next recipe) or combine 2 parts ketchup with 1 part prepared horseradish for a seafood cocktail sauce.

PUMPKIN PESTO

Featured recipe in Cooking for Fertility DVD with Tiffany Pollard and Kathryn Flynn

Pumpkin seeds are a good source of omega fatty acids and zinc, both essential for conception, hormone balance, sperm production and proper immune function. Garlic and basil vitalize the energy flow to alleviate PMS, blood clotting and fibroids, and to release stuck emotions.

Yields: 1 1/2 cup pesto

2 cups fresh basil

1 cup kale

1/2 cup pumpkin seeds

1/2 cup extra virgin olive oil

3 garlic cloves, finely minced

Juice of 1/2 a fresh lemon

Optional: For a creamier texture, add 1/2 avocado, peeled and cored Blend ingredients in food processor, using lemon juice to achieve desired consistency. Serve with shrimp cocktail, or use as a pizza or pasta sauce.

FAJITA NACHOS

This simple Mexican snack offers optimal benefits for fertility. Enjoy corn chips, a wheat-free alternative, with black beans to fortify reproductive function and with broccoli for proper hormone metabolism. Serve with guacamole and salsa (see recipes next pages).

Serves 4-6
Cooking time: 25-30 minutes, 300 degrees

1/2 onion, chopped

1/2 cup red and green peppers, sliced

1 clove garlic, minced

1/2 cup broccoli, finely chopped

1 teaspoon fajita spice

2 tablespoons extra virgin olive oil

1 bag blue corn tortilla chips

1/2 cup black beans (canned are fine)

1/2 cup goat cheese, crumbled, or almond cheese

Sauté onions, peppers, garlic, broccoli, fajita spice and olive oil over medium heat until tender. Line a baking dish with a thin layer of tortilla chips. Add a layer of black beans, followed by a layer of the onion, pepper and garlic mixture. Finally, add cheese and bake at 300 degrees for 25-30 minutes. If you have chosen to use almond cheese, please note that it does not melt as well as regular cheese. Serve on a platter with sides of guacamole and salsa.

MEXICAN SALSA

Tomatoes are cooling and nourish the adrenals, reproductive organs and kidneys, the organs most drained by the modern environment. Though tomatoes are acidic, they produce an alkalizing reaction in the body and help purify the blood. The warmer ingredients neutralize the tomato's cooling effects.

Yields: 1 cup

1 medium tomato, diced

1 clove garlic, pressed

3 green chilies, minced

2-3 green onions, chopped

6 sprigs cilantro, finely chopped

Juice of 1 fresh lime

1/4 cup water

Gently pulse all ingredients in a food processor. Serve on nachos, fajitas or corn tortilla chips.

GUACAMOLE

Avocados are 80% monounsaturated fat and provide a good serving of protein, both necessary for building blood and supporting reproductive function. As an added benefit, avocados support beautiful skin and provide healthful fats that, contrary to claims of low-fat diets, are often the key to lasting weight loss. They are rich in copper and lecithin, the former promoting red blood cell production and the latter enhancing brain function.[28]

Yields: 1 1/2 to 2 cups

6 medium-sized ripe avocados, peeled and pitted

1/2 cup Mexican salsa

Juice of 1/2 a fresh lemon

Mash avocados and add in salsa. Serve with blue corn tortilla chips and nachos.

DARK LEAFY GREEN WRAPS

Steamed or cooked veggies are generally easier to digest than raw ones. Chew any raw vegetable extra well to aid with digestion. The purple and green vegetables in this recipe support detoxification of the liver, which is often taxed by its many roles in balancing hormones, emotions, blood and stress.

Serves 2-4

10 romaine, chard, kale or collard-green leaves

Filling

1 carrot, shredded

1/2 cup purple cabbage, shredded

1/2 radish, shredded

1/2 cup slivered almonds

1/2 cup bean sprouts

1/2 cup alfalfa sprouts

2 cooked chicken breasts, cubed

Braggs Liquid Aminos for dipping

Place fillings in small bowls on the counter and encourage diners to create their own spring rolls using the leaves as wrappers. Consider serving with additional dressings, such as raita and hummus.

HUMMUS

Garbanzo beans contain more iron than any other legume, an important ingredient for building blood if you have heavy periods, which can lead to iron deficiency anemia; or if you have conditions where your bleeding is light in color or scanty. They are also a good source of healthy fats and delicious for spreading on sandwiches and rice crackers.

Yields: 2 cups

2 cups cooked garbanzo beans (also called chickpeas) – canned is fine

1 tablespoon black sesame tahini (sesame seed paste)

1 tablespoon extra virgin olive oil

Juice of 1/2 a fresh lemon

2 garlic cloves, minced

2 tablespoons fresh cilantro

1/4 teaspoon turmeric

Combine garbanzo beans, black sesame tahini, olive oil, lemon juice, garlic and cilantro in a food processor. Pulse until smooth. Transfer to a serving bowl, garnish with turmeric and chill. Serve with wedges of toasted spelt bread, raw vegetable sticks or pickles.

SUSHI ROLLS

Seaweeds are a flavorful way to introduce healthy minerals, vitamins, amino acids, calcium, iodine and iron into the diet. In Healing with Whole Foods, Paul Pitchford points out that people have drawn on sea algae "for thousands of years for their ability to prolong life, prevent disease, and impart beauty and health for happier and longer lives." To partake in the benefits of seaweeds, grind dulse in a food processor, place in a shaker and use as an alternative to table salt.

Yields: 4 rolls

4 sheets nori

Filling

2 cups brown rice, warm (see cooking whole grains in break the fast)

4 tablespoons rice vinegar

2 tablespoons toasted black sesame seeds

1/4 cup cucumber, diced

1/2 an avocado, thinly sliced

Wheat free tamari sauce for dipping, as desired

Gluten free wasabi, if desired

Pickled ginger to garnish the plate

Add rice vinegar to warm, cooked rice and stir in black sesame seeds. Combine cucumber and avocado. Place nori on a bamboo mat, and add 1/2 cup of rice mixture and 1/4 cup of filling. Roll and press to seal. Slice into desired thickness.

ROASTED GARLIC ON GOAT BRIE

Garlic builds immunity and healthy intestinal flora and clears toxins. It is a warming food that can move stuck conditions such as stagnated blood, clotting, fibroids and premenstrual tension.

Serves 6-8
Cooking Time: 35 minutes, 400 degrees then 250 degrees

1 bulb of garlic (or already prepared, peeled garlic cloves)

1 wheel goat brie

For fresh garlic: Preheat oven to 400 degrees. Cut the top off the garlic bulb, drizzle olive oil on top and roast for 30 minutes. Remove garlic and squeeze cloves from the roasted bulb and crush.

If using prepared peeled garlic: Sauté over medium heat with olive oil until tender, and mash.

In 250 degree oven, warm the goat brie wheel for 5 minutes. Place the crushed or mashed garlic on top of cheese wheel. Serve with green apple slices and wheat-free crackers.

TURKEY MEATBALLS WITH PINEAPPLE SAUCE

"Melatonin, a hormone produced by the pineal gland, is said to reduce stress, boost immunity, deepen sleep and promote longevity."[29] According to Chinese medicine, ample melatonin production improves the performance of the kidneys and adrenals, the paired organs of the reproductive system. Supplementing with melatonin, however, can disrupt estrogen function. Turkey contains tryptophan, a natural precursor that enhances your own melatonin production. By eating foods with tryptophan and B vitamins, you can reduce the impact of stress and replenish all aspects of the Kidney system. Pineapple contains bromelain, an enzyme believed to bolster implantation.

Yields: 12-16 meatballs
Cooking time: 30-35 minutes, 350 degrees

1/2 cup broccoli

1/2 cup onion

2 garlic cloves

1 lb organic ground turkey meat

2 eggs or egg replacer

1 1/2 cups wheat-free bread crumbs

1 teaspoon Herb de Provence

1 teaspoon extra virgin olive oil (for baking pan)

Place broccoli, onion and garlic in a food processor and blend thoroughly. Combine turkey and eggs or egg substitute with bread crumbs. Add minced vegetables and seasoning, and roll into bite-sized balls. Bake at 350 degrees on a greased baking pan for 30-35 minutes. Serve on a platter with toothpicks and pineapple sauce. Use leftovers with pesto pasta (Main Attraction).

Pineapple Sauce

Yields: 3/4 cup

1/2 cup fresh pineapple, chopped

1/2 cup agave nectar

2 tablespoons Dijon mustard

In a medium saucepan, combine pineapple, agave nectar and mustard and bring to a boil. Allow sauce to simmer for several minutes until thickened.

SESAME MOCHI BALLS

Nettles build the blood and are useful tonics for stimulating menses in cases of amenorrhea or delayed menstrual cycles due to blood deficiency. The rice is simmered slowly in ample water, which is helpful for nourishing the reproductive organs. This recipe is adapted from *Healing with Whole Foods* by Paul Pitchford.

Yields: 1/2 pound
Cooking time: 2 hours

1 1/2 cups sweet rice (purchase at Asian food store)

3 cups water

2 teaspoons dried nettles

1/2 cup black sesame seeds and/or coconut flakes

Simmer rice uncovered in water over low heat for approximately two hours. In the last 30 minutes, add dried nettles. Remove rice and pound with a wooden mallet until a paste is formed. Create balls and roll in black sesame seeds and coconut mixture, if desired. Serve fresh or lightly pan-fried in olive oil over medium heat.

Simmer with Soup

- The reproductive organs benefit from foods simmered slowly in water. In Chinese medicine, water is the element that corresponds to the kidneys, adrenals, and reproductive organs. So soup is an ideal meal for nourishing fertility.
- When adding vegetables to soups, choose an array of colorful, seasonal, organic vegetables (locally grown when possible).
- Always use organic, hormone-free meat products.
- Legumes provide a balanced serving of protein, fat and carbohydrates, as well as abundant potassium, calcium, iron, and B vitamins.[30]
- In any of the broth soup recipes add 1/8 cup of dang gui (angelica) to tonify the blood and/or 1/8 cup of huang qi (astralagus) to tonify the qi.
- Adding seaweed while cooking any type of soup increases mineral intake.

WHITE BEAN STEW

This soup combines warming and cooling ingredients. Onion, garlic, and chicken help to build qi and move stagnant energy. Spinach, rich in chlorophyll, combines with tomatoes to fortify and purify the blood.[31] To modify this dish's heating effects, use less garlic and onion and replace chicken with brown rice.

Serves 4
Cooking time: 60 minutes

3 cloves garlic

1/2 cup onion, chopped

1 tablespoon extra virgin olive oil

1 tablespoon thyme

2 cups cannellini or aduki beans, pre-cooked

32 ounces organic chicken stock or veggie stock

4 whole stewed tomatoes

8 ounces spinach

Optional: 1 cup roasted chicken (main attraction) or brown rice

Sea salt or dulse flakes to taste

Sauté garlic and onions in olive oil until softened. Add thyme and cannellini or aduki beans. Slowly stir in chicken stock. The longer you allow this soup to simmer, the better it tastes. Finish by adding stewed tomatoes and spinach, until wilted.

BLACK BEAN SOUP

In TCM, black beans are used to fortify the kidneys and enhance fertility. These nourishing legumes help to resolve symptoms like low back pain and low libido while replenishing your deepest reserves.[32]

Serves 4
Cooking time: 60 minutes

3 cups black beans, precooked
1 cup onion, chopped
3 garlic cloves
1/2 cup carrot, sliced
1/2 cup celery, chopped
1 cup yam or sweet potatoes, cubed
1/2 cup bell pepper, chopped
1/2 teaspoon five spice
1 teaspoon cumin
3 tablespoons extra virgin olive oil
32 ounces organic chicken stock or veggie stock
1 cup water
2 inch piece of kombu
1 avocado, diced to garnish
Sea salt or dulse flakes to taste

In a large pot, sauté garlic, onion, carrot, celery, yam, bell pepper, spices and olive oil over medium heat, uncovered. Add chicken stock, water, beans and kombu. Bring to boil, and reduce to simmer for at least one hour, then transfer 1 cup portions to a warmed blender and pulse until smooth.

LONGEVITY SOUP

In China, the broth from broken bone soup is referred to as longevity soup. This soup replenishes your very essence and builds the blood with the valuable omega-3 fatty acid DHA. This soup is also recommended for breastfeeding mothers to support development of the baby's nerves, cells, tissues, and bones.[33]

Yields: 4 liters
Cooking time: 5-6 hours

6 organic beef bones

2 onions, chopped

2 carrots, sliced

2 celery stalks, sliced

2 bay leaves

1 bunch parsley stems

1/2 teaspoon black pepper

1/2 teaspoon dulse

1 tablespoon lemon juice

6 quarts cold water

Combine all ingredients in a large pot and bring to a boil. Reduce and simmer uncovered for five or more hours. Remove bones and save the broth, using as a base for other soups or to sip on throughout the day.

BUTTERNUT SQUASH BISQUE

Squash is a beneficial source of Vitamin A. Cooling and replenishing in nature, it helps resolve inflammatory conditions.[34] Ginger is a good digestive aid, while the warming properties of onions and nutmeg encourage energy flow.

Serves 4
Cooking time: 40 minutes

1 tablespoon extra virgin olive oil
2-3 pounds butternut squash, peeled and diced
3 large carrots, chopped
1 medium onion, chopped
1/2 teaspoon nutmeg
1 tablespoon fresh ginger, minced
32 ounces organic vegetable broth
1 bunch parsley
Sea salt or dulse flakes to taste

Heat olive oil in a large pot, and sauté squash, carrots, onion, nutmeg and ginger until lightly browned. Add vegetable broth, and bring to a boil. Simmer uncovered for 40 minutes, until vegetables are tender. Puree soup in blender until smooth and creamy. Garnish with parsley and serve.

CREAM OF VEGETABLE SOUP

All the healthy vitamins and antioxidants in these vegetables will purify and balance your entire system.

Serves 4
Cooking time: 50 minutes

2 leeks, white part only, chopped

2 garlic cloves

1/2 cup water

1 medium carrot, chopped

1 celery stalk, sliced

2 cups canned tomatoes

1 1/2 + 1/2 cup almond or goat milk

2 teaspoons arrowroot powder

1/2 teaspoon salt

1/4 teaspoon pepper

1/2 teaspoon thyme

1 bay leaf

2 teaspoons tomato paste

Combine leeks, garlic, and water. Simmer until leeks are soft. Add carrots and celery. Simmer five more minutes. Add tomato and 1 1/2 cup of milk. Simmer until mixture comes to a boil. At same time combine the other 1/2 cup of milk with the arrowroot powder, whisking until smooth. Then whisk this thickener into the soup. Add seasonings and tomato paste.. Simmer 30 minutes, uncovered, stirring frequently. Preheat blender with hot water, then empty. Pour soup mixture in, and blend until smooth.

FERTILITY STEW

This nourishing soup is created specifically for fertility with purifying garlic and onions, mineral-rich seaweed, cruciferous vegetables, calming brown rice, yams to stimulate the ovaries, and tofu for cooling replenishment. With balanced grains, vegetables and protein, this soup makes a complete meal.

Serves 4
Cooking time: 40 minutes

2 teaspoons extra virgin olive oil

3 cloves garlic, minced

1 portobello mushroom, sliced thinly

2 leeks, chopped

2 celery stalks

1 small head cabbage

6 plum tomatoes, diced

32 ounces organic chicken or vegetable stock

1 yam, cubed

1 piece dried kelp

1 6-ounce package tofu or 2 cups shrimp

1 cup black beans, cooked

1 cup brown rice, cooked

1/2 cup broccoli, chopped

In a large pot heat olive oil, and sauté garlic, mushrooms, leeks, and celery until browned. Add cabbage and tomatoes, simmering for five minutes. Add broth, yam, and kelp. Bring to a boil. After 10 minutes reduce heat, and add tofu or shrimp, black beans, rice, and broccoli. When broccoli becomes bright green, soup is ready.

GAZPACHO

This cooling soup with a bite is a good choice for a hot summer day.

Serves 4

1/2 cup red wine vinegar

1/2 cup extra virgin olive oil

6 large ripe tomatoes with juice, chopped

1 1/2 cups tomato juice

2 red bell peppers, cored, seeded, and coarsely chopped

2 onions, coarsely chopped

2 cloves garlic

2 large cucumbers, coarsely chopped

Sea salt or dulse flakes to taste

1/2 cup fresh dill

Place all ingredients in a food processor or blender, and combine until smooth. Serve at room temperature.

GREEN PUREE

Green foods are the richest chlorophyll sources, and in TCM the color green is associated with the spring, a time of renewal. Chlorophyll purifies and reduces inflammation; it is known as "the blood of plant life."[35]

Serves 4
Cooking time: 40 minutes

1/2 cup broccoli, chopped

3 cups leafy greens, chopped

2 teaspoons extra virgin olive oil

2 leeks, chopped

2 zucchini, sliced

3 celery stalks, sliced

1 small onion

16 ounces of organic vegetable broth

16 ounces of water

Steam broccoli and leafy greens until tender. In separate pot, heat olive oil, and sauté leeks, zucchini, celery and onion until softened. Add greens, vegetable broth and water and simmer for 20 minutes. Remove from heat and puree one-cup portions at a time. Return to low heat and add simmer for two hours.

CHILI

Packed with hearty bean protein and turkey's relaxing tryptophan, this is the perfect meal to warm you on a cold winter night.

Serves 4
Cooking time: 45 minutes

1 1/2 pounds ground lean organic turkey or beef

1 large can stewed tomatoes

1 red pepper, chopped

1 green pepper, chopped

1 onion, diced

1 serving chili seasoning to taste (see below)

2 cups red kidney beans, cooked (canned or pre-cooked)

2 cups black beans, cooked (canned or pre-cooked)

In a pot, brown meat thoroughly and drain fat. Add tomatoes, vegetables, chili seasoning and beans, and simmer on low heat for 30 minutes or more.

Chili seasoning

1/2 teaspoon oregano

1/2 teaspoon paprika

1/2 teaspoon cayenne

1 teaspoon cumin

1 teaspoon garlic powder

MISO

The cooling properties of tofu, spinach, and wakame make this an excellent choice to replenish a stressed system. The Japanese eat miso soup in the morning for a nutrient-rich start to the day.

Serves 2
Cooking time: 25 minutes

1 onion, diced

1 handful spinach

1 white mushroom, sliced thin

1 teaspoon extra virgin olive oil

2 cups water

1/2 cup wakame, pre-soaked and cut into pieces

1 tablespoon red miso paste

1 slice extra firm tofu, cubed

Saute onion, spinach and mushroom in olive oil; add water, wakame and miso paste, and simmer for 10 minutes. Add tofu during the last two minutes, and then serve.

CURRIED ROOT STEW

This is a grounding soup that helps us connect to our own roots – our kidneys, adrenals, and reproductive organs. It supports our sense of foundation in the world with earth-energy nourishment.

Serves 4
Cooking time: 3 hours

1 medium beet

1 medium yam

1 medium squash

1 small rutabaga

1 medium turnip

1 leek

32 ounces water or organic vegetable broth

2 teaspoons curry powder

Sea salt or dulse flakes to taste

Cut all vegetables into small cubes. Place in pot with liquid, bring to a boil, add curry powder, and reduce heat to simmer, uncovered, for three hours. Enjoy as pureed soup, or sip on broth for nourishment throughout the day.

LENTIL SOUP

Lentils are a traditional staple of India and help to increase vitality at our core, replenishing our inner reservoirs of energy at the deepest level.[36] Lentils are a great source of fiber, iron and B vitamins and also help to stabilize blood sugar levels.

Serves 4
Cooking time: 60 minutes

2 tablespoons extra virgin olive oil

3/4 cup onion, chopped

2 cloves garlic, minced

32 ounces chicken or vegetable broth

2 cups lentils

1/2 cup carrot, chopped

1/2 cup celery, chopped

1/4 teaspoon coriander

1/4 teaspoon cumin

Sea salt or dulse flakes to taste

Over medium heat, sauté olive oil, onion, and garlic in a large pot. Add chicken or vegetable stock, lentils, carrots, celery, and spices. Simmer over medium low for 40 minutes. Puree mixture in a heated blender until smooth, or leave chunky as desired. Add salt and pepper to taste, and serve hot.

CARROT GINGER SOUP

Carrots are a good source of beta-carotene and help to regulate all hormones in the body. They also support beautiful skin, clearing cases of acne, and help metabolize calcium.[37]

Serves 4
Cooking time: 40-60 minutes

2 tablespoons extra virgin olive oil

1 cup onion, chopped

2 tablespoons fresh ginger, minced

32 ounces of organic chicken or vegetable broth

1 pound bag of carrot, sliced

1 cup almond or goat milk

1/4 teaspoon cinnamon

1/4 teaspoon allspice

1/2 teaspoon arrowroot powder

Sea salt or dulse flakes to taste

Over medium heat, sauté olive oil, onion, and ginger in a large pot. Add chicken stock and carrots, bringing to a boil and simmering over medium low for 10 minutes. Add milk, spices, and arrowroot, simmering for 20 minutes more. Preheat blender with hot water; puree mixture until smooth. Add salt and pepper to taste, and serve hot.

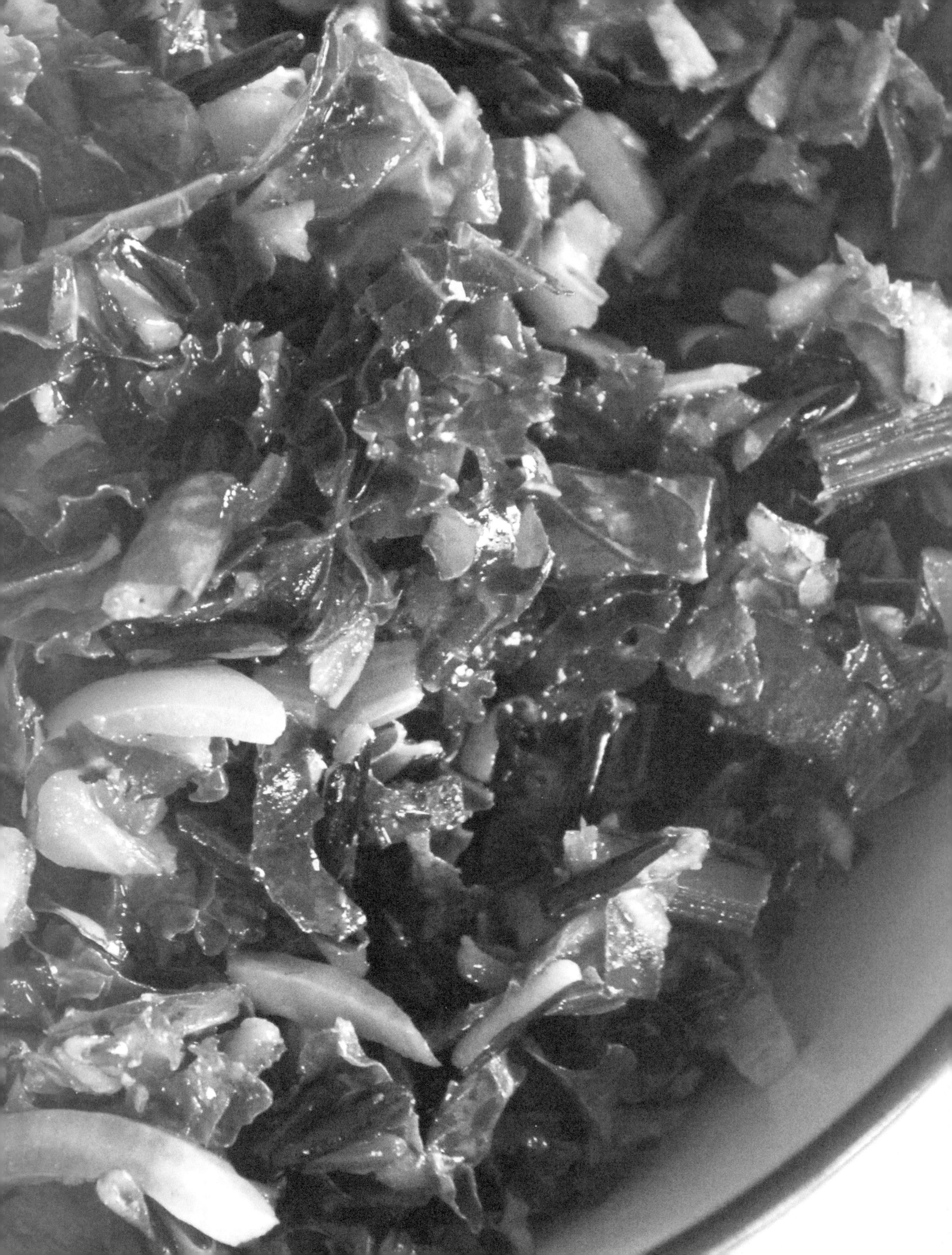

Slowly with Salad

- Raw vegetables are cleansing and detoxifying. Chew them thoroughly (at least 30 bites per chew) to help support digestive processes.
- If you have difficulty finding organic produce, soak fruit and vegetables in 1:1 water and vinegar solution to remove pesticides. Environmental toxins like pesticides have been linked to cancer and many reproductive disorders.
- Eat cooling raw vegetables in the spring and summer. Otherwise, favor steamed vegetables, especially during cooler weather. As a rule, eat salad at room temperature, rather than chilled from the refrigerator.
- Experiment with different varieties of dark leafy greens to optimize your chlorophyll intake, including kale, chard, red chard, spinach, romaine, and arugula.
- Choose freshly picked and locally grown organic vegetables whenever possible. We receive more qi/energy from foods consumed closer to their source.
- Instead of croutons, we suggest these flavorful and healthy salad sprinklings:

  Black sesame seeds
  Dulse flakes
  Pumpkin seeds
  Sunflower seeds
  Almonds
  Goji berries
  Cranberries

- For a simplified dressing, drizzle your salad with Usana Optomega oil, flaxseed oil, or extra virgin olive oil

ROASTED BEET, PISTACHIO AND PEAR SALAD

In TCM, the color red in the beet indicates its benefits to both the heart and the blood. It is helpful food for stimulating more frequent menstruation for those with longer cycles, or for treating amenorrhea.[38]

Serves 2-4
Cooking time: 45 minutes, 375 degrees

2 beets, peeled

1 cup pear, diced

1/4 cup celery

2 tablespoons pistachios, chopped

3 tablespoons lemon juice

1 tablespoon agave syrup

1/4 tablespoon white pepper

Heat oven to 375 degrees and roast cleaned beets for 45 minutes or until tender. Cool and dice. Combine beets, pear, celery and pistachios in a small bowl. In a separate bowl, whisk together lemon juice, agave syrup and white pepper. Drizzle beets with lemon juice mixture, and serve alone or with mixed greens.

COLE SLAW

Cabbage, radish and lemon support a free-flowing liver and help alleviate symptoms of pre-menstrual tension, irritability, headaches, or breast tenderness at ovulation.

Serves 4-6

3 cups red or green cabbage, thinly sliced

2 radishes, grated

1/2 cup slivered almonds

2 tablespoons black sesame seeds

Deb's Simple Cider Vinagrette

1/4 cup apple cider vinegar

1/4 cup flaxseed oil

1/4 cup Braggs amino acids

Combine cabbages, radishes, almonds and sesame seeds in a bowl. In a separate jar mix together apple cider vinegar, flaxseed oil and Braggs amino acid. Pour over salad, mix and serve.

SOUTHWESTERN BLACK BEAN SALAD

This salad contains a number of fertile foods. In TCM black beans are used to fortify the kidneys and enhance fertility.[39] Corn is a heart-nourishing grain that promotes vitality in the sexual organs.[40] Yams and sweet potatoes build up yin fluids like cervical mucus and semen and increase vital life force energy.[41]

Serves 4-6

2 ears corn

1 jalapeno pepper (optional)

1 tablespoon olive oil

4 plum tomatoes, seeded and diced

2 cloves garlic, minced

1/2 cup onion, chopped

1 1/2 cup black beans, cooked

1 medium yam baked, cooked and cubed

3 tablespoons cilantro

1/2 cup corn chips (optional)

Chipotle lime dressing

2 tablespoons extra virgin olive oil

2 tablespoons lime juice

1 tsp chipotle pepper

Sea salt or dulse flakes to taste

Brush corn and jalapeno with oil. Grill, on high heat for about five minutes. Remove skin and seeds from jalapeno, and slice kernels off cob. Combine corn, jalapeno, tomatoes, garlic and onions with black beans, yams and cilantro. Stir together with dressing. Add corn chips, if desired.

CUCUMBER, KALE AND SEAWEED SALAD

"The power of sea vegetables (seaweeds) have been drawn on for thousands of years for their ability to prolong life, prevent disease, and impart beauty and health for happier, longer lives."[42] Seaweeds build up our very essence, fortifying our inherent fertility.

Serves 4-6

3 cups kale, shredded

1/2 cup cucumber

1/2 cup wakame, soaked

1/2 cup dulse, soaked

1/4 cup red onion

1/4 cup apple

1 tablespoon black sesame seeds

Anti-inflammatory dressing

1/2 cup unsweetened pineapple juice

2 tablespoons apple cider vinegar

1 clove garlic, crushed

1 teaspoon sesame oil

Sea salt or dulse flakes to taste

Put prepared kale in a big salad bowl. Dice the cucumber, wakame, dulse, red onion, and apple, and add to kale. In a separate jar mix juice, vinegar, garlic, sesame oil, and dulse flakes. Shake well; add to vegetables, top with sesame seeds, toss and serve.

GRATEFUL GREENS

Green foods are the richest chlorophyll sources and in TCM, they are associated with the spring, a time of renewal and regeneration. Chlorophyll purifies and reduces inflammation. Chlorophyll is sometimes called "the blood of plant life."[43] Topped with raspberry vinaigrette, which is a delicious way to nourish the blood and regulate the menstrual cycle.[44]

Serves 2-4

1 portobello mushroom, sliced
1 teaspoon extra virgin olive oil
2 cups mixed greens
1 tomato, diced
1 avocado, sliced
1/4 cup walnut pieces or almond slivers
1/4 cup cranberries
1/4 cup goat feta cheese (optional)

Lightly sauté sliced mushroom in olive oil. Wash, dry, and place mixed greens in large serving bowl. Separate bowl into quarters and create wedges with each of the following ingredients: tomato, mushroom, avocado, walnuts, and cranberries. Sprinkle goat cheese in the middle. Toss with raspberry vinaigrette at the table.

Raspberry vinaigrette

1/2 cup fresh or frozen raspberries
1/4 cup extra virgin olive oil
1/4 cup balsamic vinegar
1/8 cup raspberry balsamic vinegar

Combine all four ingredients in a blender.

RED BLISS SALAD

Potatoes come from the earth and support our roots and inner yin, improving our "receptive, nurturing and compassionate nature."[45] They are a wonderful source of Vitamin C, enzymes, and minerals and are most nourishing when consumed with their skin left on. Red bliss potatoes have a lower glycemic index than most other white potatoes.

Serves 4-6

3 pounds red bliss potatoes

1/2 cup chopped parsley

6 scallions, finely sliced

Salt and pepper to taste

Mustard dressing

1/4 cup Dijon mustard

1/2 cup extra virgin olive oil

1/2 cup unsweetened pineapple juice

1/8 cup apple cider vinegar

6 fresh basil leaves, chopped

Steam potatoes with skin on for 20 minutes or until tender. In the meantime, combine mustard and olive oil in food processor. Add pineapple juice, vinegar, and basil leaves. Blend until texture is creamy. Once potatoes have cooled, cube, and place in large bowl with parsley and scallions. Add dressing and serve.

CAESAR SALAD

This recipe combines a traditional Caesar salad with sardines, often an acquired taste. This fish is beneficial to fertility as a source of protein that builds the yin reserves and supports blood circulation.[46]

Serves 4-6

1 head romaine lettuce

2 ounces sardines (optional)

Croutons

1 tablespoon clarified butter/ghee

1 clove fresh garlic, crushed

3 slices spelt bread

Garlic dressing

1/2 cup extra virgin olive oil

2 tablespoons red wine vinegar

1 clove fresh garlic, crushed

1 lemon, juiced

1/4 tablespoon ground mustard

1 teaspoon Worcestershire sauce

Sauté ghee and garlic over medium heat. Cut spelt bread into bite-size cubes, and sauté until golden brown. Put aside. Tear lettuce into bite-size pieces, and place in mixing bowl. In a separate bowl whisk together oil, vinegar, garlic, lemon juice, mustard and Worcestershire sauce. Add dressing to lettuce, top with sardines and croutons, and serve.

GREEK SALAD

A mix of chunky vegetables, topped with olives' omega goodness and delicious goat feta.

Serves 4-6

2 cucumbers, halved and sliced
1 red onion, thickly sliced
2 large tomatoes, chopped
1 cup crumbled goat feta cheese
1 can pitted black olives

Oregano dressing

6 tablespoons extra virgin olive oil
2 tablespoons balsamic vinegar
1 teaspoon dried oregano
1 lemon, juiced
Sea salt or dulse flakes to taste

Combine cucumber, red onion, tomatoes, goat feta, and olives in a large mixing bowl. In a separate bowl, whisk together olive oil, balsamic, oregano, and lemon juice. Add dressing to vegetables, and transfer into a salad bowl to serve.

SPINACH SALAD

Spinach is rich in iron and chlorophyll, helping to build and purify the blood. This salad provides a good dose of omegas with the walnuts and flaxseed oil. Steaming the spinach in this salad preserves the taste and adds to its digestibility.[47]

Serves 4-6

12 ounces spinach, fresh or lightly steamed

1 cup strawberries, sliced

1/3 cup walnuts or pinenuts

3 tablespoons goat cheese

3 strips turkey bacon, cooked and cut into strips

Omega pesto dressing

1/2 cup fresh basil

1/4 cup kale

1/4 cup pumpkin seeds

1/8 cup extra virgin olive oil

1 garlic cloves, finely minced

Juice of 1/4 lemon

1/2 avocado, peeled and cored

Combine spinach, strawberries, nuts, goat cheese, and turkey bacon in a bowl. Blend dressing ingredients in food processor, using lemon juice to achieve desired consistency.

PASTA BRUSCHETTA

Experiment with alternatives to traditional white pasta. Not only does this avoid the heavy glycemic hit from white pasta, but it reaps the benefits of whatever whole grains you use. For instance, brown rice is rich in antioxidants and heartcalming properties, while quinoa is the grain with the most protein.

Serves 4-6

4 quarts water

2 cups brown rice or quinoa spirals

1/2 cup arugula

2 chicken breasts, cooked, or 1 cup shrimp, peeled and cooked

8 cherry tomatoes, halved

1/4 cup fresh basil, chopped

1/4 cup goat feta (optional)

4 tablespoons extra virgin olive oil

Salt and pepper to taste

In a large saucepan, bring water to a boil. Add pasta, reduce to medium heat, and continue to boil for directed time, until al dente. Drain well, and place in a serving bowl. Toss with arugula, chicken or shrimp, tomatoes, basil, feta and olive oil. Salt and pepper as desired. Serve hot or cold.

WALDORF SALAD

Apples are cooling in nature and have the capacity to nourish our yin, which is often depleted by stress and the fast pace of our lives. Apples benefit low blood sugar conditions and emotional depression.[48] In this recipe, apples combine with the omega goodness of walnuts and a delicious dose of full-fat goat dairy dressing.

Serves 2-4

1/2 cup walnuts, chopped

1/2 cup celery, thinly sliced

1/4 cup of cranberries or raisins

1 red or green apple, cored and chopped

1 cup mixed greens

Light goat dressing

1/2 cup extra virgin olive oil

3/4 cup goat milk

2 teaspoons agave nectar

1 teaspoon apple cider vinegar

1/2 teaspoon Dijon mustard

1 tsp arrowroot powder

Combine walnuts, celery, cranberries, and apple. In a blender combine dressing ingredients and mix on low until combined. Serve on top of mixed greens.

QUINOA TABOULI

Quinoa, a seed, is often referred to as "the mother of grains." It contains 16 per cent more protein that any other grain, warming you from the inside out. This plant-based protein also provides manganese, magnesium and iron, as well as all nine essential amino acids.[49] Parsley is also rich in benefits. With Vitamin A, chlorophyll, calcium, sodium and magnesium, it is known to fortify the adrenals, a paired organ of the reproductive system.[50]

Serves 4-6

2 cups water

1 cup quinoa, soaked and rinsed

1/2 cup edamame beans

1 tomato, diced

1/2 cucumber, sliced

6 black olives, sliced

Lemon vinaigrette

1/2 teaspoon minced chives

1/2 teaspoon minced parsley

3 tablespoons lemon juice

1 tablespoon wheat-free tamari sauce

Combine water and quinoa in a pot. Cover, bring to a boil, and simmer for 20 minutes. Steam edamame for 1 minute. Put edamame in a bowl, and mix with tomato, cucumber and black olives. Add quinoa and toss gently with lemon vinaigrette. Serve warm or cool to room temperature.

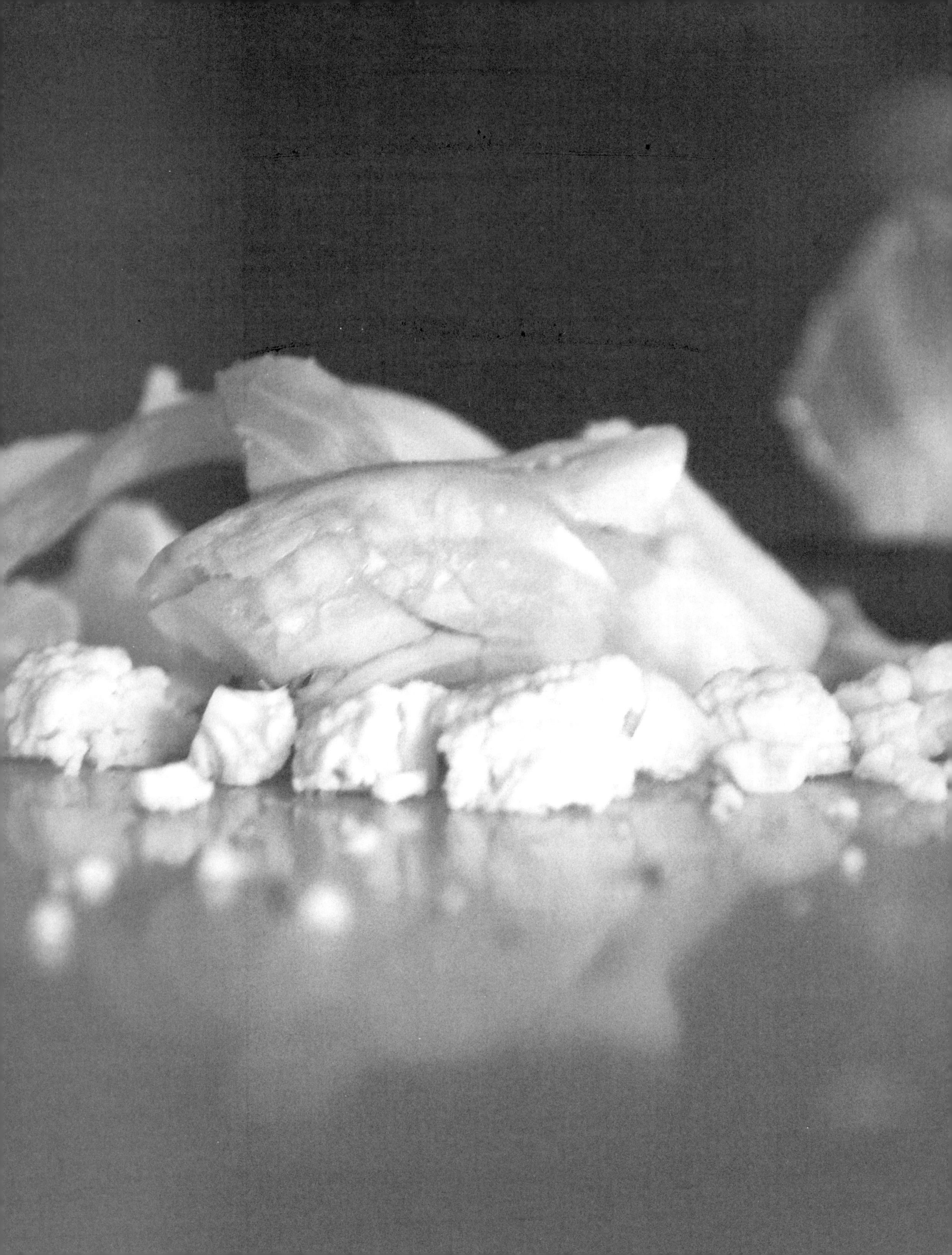

On the Side

- Load up on veggies and whole grains. The Chinese eat 70 per cent more fiber and 30 per cent more carbohydrates than Americans do, and one-third of the protein. China boasts a significantly healthier population with a lower incidence of heart disease, cancer, and osteoporosis than the U.S.[51]
- Grains and vegetables contain important nutrients, known to boost cell regeneration and proper immune function, support neuro-transmitter function, and reduce inflammation.[52]
- Eat cooked foods to support optimum digestion, trusting that with proper cooking you will still receive plenty of the nutrients. Cooked foods build qi and contribute to an overall sense of grounding, while raw foods tend to activate the mind.[53]
- "Proper cooking methods (not overcooking) can preserve well over 90 percent of [a vegetable's] nutrients. Although some Vitamin C is destroyed by heat, cooking breaks down the cellulose structure, making other nutrients more accessible than they would be otherwise."[54]
- "Serve vegetables with grain for complete nourishment. In general, grains build, while vegetables cleanse the body of toxins, and purify and renew the blood. The combination is healing and soothing."[55]

SIMPLE BEANS AND LEGUMES

Beans are sweet and support digestion, especially when their complex sugars are broken down through soaking. To simplify the process, use a 2 1/2 quart crock pot with 2 cups of dry beans. Soak for several hours or overnight, and then discard the soaking water. Add water or broth with seasoning and cook for six to eight hours, while at work or overnight. To prepare beans in the traditional manner using the chart below, soak them overnight. Then place water or broth and beans in a pot, and bring to a boil for 15 minutes, removing excess foam from top of water. Cover, and simmer for recommended cooking time. Add spices to taste, and seaweed for additional minerals. Serve as a side dish for breakfast, lunch, or dinner.

Cooking and Serving Instructions

1 cup of dry beans	Water or broth	Cooking time	Characteristics	How to serve	TCM Benefits
Aduki	2-4 cups	2 hours	Small red beans originating in Asia, with a strong texture and flavor.	Vegetarian burgers, soups, rice dishes	Blood deficiency, blood stasis, heat, dampness, kidney yang deficiency
Black	2-4 cups	4 hours	Medium, sweet taste, popular in the Caribbean islands.	Spread, burgers, Mexican dishes, mashed	Spleen Qi deficiency, kidney yin deficiency
Garbanzo	2-4 cups	6 hours	Pale yellow with a firm, "nut-like" taste, originating in the Middle East.	Hummus, Mediterrane an dishes	Spleen Qi deficiency
Kidney	2-4 cups	4 hours	Deep red, commonly found in the US, with a robust flavor and texture.	Chili, soups, salad	Dampness, Kidney deficiency
Lima	2-4 cups	3 hours	Large greenish white with a creamy texture, often consumed South America	Soups, salads	Excess heat, blood stasis
Lentils	2-4 cups	1½ hours	Found in a range of colors yellow, orange, green and black- this legume	Soup, sprouted loaves, mashed	Spleen qi deficiency, kidney yang deficiency
Mung	2-4 cups	1½ hours	An asian bean, light yellow in color used often in Ayurvedic cooking for its many healing properties and digestibility	Dahl, Asian dishes	Kidney yin deficiency, excess heat

MOROCCAN PILAF

Pepper, cloves, cardamom and onions help restore hormonal balance by clearing stagnant conditions, including PMS, irritability and cramping. The apricots and goji berries balance those ingredients with their yin-nourishing properties, helping to replenish our deepest reserves.

Serves 4-6
Cooking time: 50-60 minutes

1 tablespoon extra virgin olive oil

1 medium onion, chopped

2/3 cup cashews, halved

1/3 cup goji berries

3 cups cooked brown rice

1 cup dried apricots

1/4 teaspoon ground cinnamon

1/4 teaspoon turmeric

1/4 teaspoon cracked black pepper

1/8 teaspoon cardamom

1/8 teaspoon ground cloves

1/2 cup organic chicken or vegetable broth

In large skillet, sauté onion in olive oil over medium heat. Add cashews and goji berries; sauté 2-3 minutes until nuts begin to brown and goji berries plump. Add rice, apricots, and all the spices. Stir in broth. Heat and serve.

BROCCOLI WITH OYSTER SAUCE

Broccoli is rich in cancer-preventing phytochemicals and contains high levels of vitamin A, vitamin C, sulfur, iron, and B vitamins. It promotes bright eyes, the organ paired with the liver.[56] Oysters, a commonly known aphrodisiac, help build blood and yin. They often are used to overcome nervous conditions and indecision.[57]

Serves 4-6
Cooking time: 15 minutes

2 heads broccoli

1 teaspoon olive oil

1 spring onion, finely sliced

1 small piece of ginger

2 tablespoons corn flour

1/4 cup chopped walnuts

Sauce:

1/2 cup organic chicken or veggie stock

1 1/2 tablespoons oyster sauce

1/2 tablespoon Japanese cooking wine

1/2 teaspoon wheat-free tamari

1/2 teaspoon pepper

Steam broccoli 3-4 minutes. Heat oil, add onion and ginger, and stir-fry. Add the sauce and broccoli, and stir to combine. When sauce simmers, add corn flour, and stir to coat broccoli. Add walnuts and serve immediately.

COCONUT RICE WITH PEPITAS

Black rice is a delicious grain that turns indigo when cooked. Its high iron content combines beautifully with coconut milk and refreshing mango, known to build yin fluids including semen and cervical mucous.[58] This dish can be served hot or cold.

Serves 4-6
Cooking time: 50-60 minutes

2 cups black rice, uncooked (can use brown or red varieties)

3 cups coconut milk

2 1/2 cups water

1/2 cup shredded coconut

1/2 teaspoon extra virgin olive oil

2 tablespoons pepitas (pumpkin) seeds

1 mango, chopped (optional)

In a pot, bring water, rice and coconut milk to a boil, stirring frequently. Reduce heat to medium low, add shredded coconut and simmer, covered, for 40 minutes. Once liquid has evaporated, remove from heat and allow to sit covered for 10 minutes. Stir-fry rice pumpkins seeds with olive oil and add on top. Option: Serve leftovers cold, and add mango for great taste.

PINEAPPLE GINGER FRIED RICE

Antioxidant-rich brown rice is a staple side. Here it is combined with anti-inflammatory pineapple and ginger to nourish the body and prepare for conception.

Yields 4-6
Cooking time: 50-60 minutes

2 cups cooked brown rice (you can substitute leftover black rice also)

2 tablespoons extra virgin olive oil

1 tbsp crushed ginger

1/2 cup fresh or frozen pineapple

Heat olive oil in a skillet, add rice and reduce to medium heat. Add in ginger and pineapple and cook on medium-low heat for an additional 5-10 minutes.

YAM FRIES

Combine the warming qualities of rosemary, thyme, sage and parsley with sweet yams for a heart-healthy alternative to fast-food fries. A recent study by Harvard Medical School has shown that the trans fats found in a small serving of commercial French fries are enough to affect fertility.[59]

Serves 4
Cooking time: 45-60 minutes, 400 degrees

2 medium yams, cut into 1/8 -inch strips

2 tablespoons extra virgin olive oil

1/2 teaspoon parsley

1/4 teaspoon sage

1/4 teaspoon thyme

1/2 teaspoon rosemary

Sea salt or dulse flakes to taste

Preheat oven to 400 degrees. Slice sweet potato into circles or thin strips. Baste with olive oil, and add spices. Place a single layer on baking sheet, and cook for 45 minutes or until tender inside and crisp outside.

COCONUT DAL

Dal is a thick spicy bean dish commonly prepared in India and Pakistan. Cumin, turmeric, ginger, garlic and coriander will warm you from the inside out and balance the deep nourishing qualities of mung beans and coconut milk. Mung beans are often used in Chinese cuisine to detoxify the body and tame impatience. Lentils increase blood flow, supporting our adrenals and inner vitality.[60] Take care with this dish if you have heat signs like hot flashes or night sweats.

Serves 4-6
Cooking time: 12 hours pre-soaking + 40-60 minutes

1 cup mung beans or lentils

2 1/2 cups water

1 cup coconut milk

1/4 teaspoon turmeric

1/4 teaspoon coriander

2 cloves garlic

1/2 teaspoon ginger

2 tablespoons extra virgin olive oil

1/2 teaspoon cumin

1 small onion

Presoak mung beans overnight. Rinse and drain. Bring water and coconut milk to a boil with beans, turmeric, coriander, ginger, and garlic. Cover, and simmer for 30 minutes. In the meantime, heat olive oil with cumin briefly, being careful not to burn the spice, and add onion, cooking until golden brown. Add dal mixture to skillet. Heat on low until dal thickens.

RATATOUILLE

Eggplant, a rich source of bioflavanoids, is an ideal treatment for stagnant blood in the uterus. On an emotional level, it is believed to assist in resolving repressed emotion in both the uterus and liver. Due to its hemostatic qualities, do not consume eggplant in abundance during pregnancy.[61]

Serves 6-8

2 tablespoons extra virgin olive oil

1 small onion, thinly sliced

2 cloves garlic, crushed and minced

1 eggplant, cubed

2 green peppers, chopped

4 large tomatoes, diced

3 zucchini, thinly sliced

1 teaspoon basil

1/2 teaspoon oregano

1/4 teaspoon thyme

Fresh parsley

In large skillet (at least 14") heat olive oil, reduce to medium, add onions and garlic and saute until tender. Add eggplant and peppers. Cook for 10 minutes. Add tomatoes, zucchini, herbs, and cook on low for 15 minutes. Garnish with parsley.

ROASTED ROSEMARY ROOTS

Root vegetables "grow in cold climates and contain minerals and other elements that make it possible to survive in harsh weather and under snow. When eating, we take on their qualities and build resistance to cool weather and disease."[62]

Serves 6-8
Cooking time: 40 minutes, 400 degrees

2 beets

1 small eggplant

1 leek

1 turnips

1 sweet potato

1 rutabaga

2-3 tablespoons extra virgin olive oil

1 clove garlic, minced

1 tablespoon fresh rosemary

Flaxseed oil to taste

Preheat oven to 400 degrees. Peel and chop vegetables into bite-sized pieces. Toss with olive oil, garlic and rosemary, and lay flat on baking pan. Bake for 40 minutes, until all vegetables are tender. Drizzle with flaxseed oil and serve.

CRUCIFEROUS CRUNCH

"Cruciferous vegetables contain di-indolymethane (DIM), a compound that stimulates more efficient use of estrogen by increasing the metabolism of estradiol (one form of estrogen produced in the body). Excess estrogen is associated with breast pain, weight gain, breast and uterine cancer, moodiness and low libido."[63]

Serves 4-6
Cooking time: 45-60 minutes, 400 degrees

1 1/2 cups cauliflower

1 1/2 cups broccoli

1/4 cup extra virgin olive oil

Sea salt or dulse flakes to taste

Preheat over to 400 degrees. Toss cauliflower and broccoli in a bowl with olive oil and sea salt. Place in the oven, and roast for 45-60 minutes.

CAULI-MASH

Here's another healthy, delicious way to consume the cruciferous vegetables that metabolize excess estrogens. That frees the liver to support its many functions including metabolizing emotions, hormones and blood. Sprinkle with turmeric for further liver detoxification and anti-inflammatory properties.

Serves 4-6
Cooking time: 10 minutes

3 cups cauliflower, steamed

1 tablespoon clarified butter/ghee

1 garlic clove

1 tablespoon goat milk

1/4 teaspoon turmeric (optional)

Steam cauliflower 5-10 minutes, until tender. In a food processor, blend with ghee, garlic and goat milk. Sprinkle with turmeric and serve as you would the traditional version of mashed potatoes.

HAWAIIAN CARROTS

Carrots contain abundant beta-carotene and help alkalize the blood.[64] Pineapple contains bromelain, an enzyme believed to bolster implantation.

Serves 2-4
Cooking time: 30 minutes, 375 degrees

1/4 macadamia nut oil

1/2 cup fresh pineapple

1 cup carrots

Preheat oven to 375 degrees. Blend oil and fresh pineapple on medium speed for five minutes. Toss with carrots, place in casserole dish, and bake for 30 minutes or until tender.

GINGER SESAME ASPARAGUS

Asparagus encourages yin receptivity and compassion in overly aggressive men or women. It is known to enhance fertility and soften difficult menses.[65]

Serves 2-4
Cooking time: 5-10 minutes

1 pound asparagus

1 teaspoon extra virgin olive oil

1/4 teaspoon sesame seeds

1 teaspoon ginger, grated

Sea salt or dulse flakes to taste

Wash, and break off ends of asparagus. Toss asparagus with olive oil, sesame seeds, ginger and salt, and then sauté on medium heat in a large skillet for three minutes on medium-high heat, cooking until tender.

LOADED YAMS WITH MIGHTY GREENS

An excellent alternative to the traditional baked potato. Yams are a colorful, low-glycemic choice and with the turkey bacon can be enjoyed as a full meal.

Serves 2-4
Cooking time: 60 minutes, 375 degrees

2 medium yams

1 tablespoon extra virgin olive oil

1/4 cup red and/or green peppers, sliced

1/4 cup red onion, sliced

1 cup mighty greens (any combination of kale, nettles, chard and spinach)

2 tablespoons garlic, crushed

2 strips turkey bacon, cooked and sliced

Heat oven to 375 degrees. Bake yams for 45-60 minutes until soft. Toward the end of the baking period, sauté olive oil, peppers, greens, onion, and garlic on medium heat. Slice open yams, and top with vegetable mixture. Top with turkey bacon bits if desired.

SWEET YAM AND WALNUT CASSEROLE

A sweet omega-3 side dish, delightful served with Tri-Tip Roast (Main Attraction) and Loaded Yams with Mighty Greens (previous page).

Serves 6-8
Cooking time: 60-70 minutes, 375 degrees

8 medium yams

1 1/2 cups walnuts

2 tablespoons agave nectar

Heat oven to 375 degrees. Bake yams for 45-60 minutes until soft. Cover walnuts with agave nectar. Arrange on baking sheet, and cook for last 10 minutes with yams. Remove skin from yams, mash in casserole dish, and add crushed candied walnuts.

SAUERKRAUT

"Raw, saltless sauerkraut is an excellent food for regenerating the intestines. It harmonizes the digestion by balancing the secretions of the stomach, helps in the formation of enzymes and vitamins, strengthens the function of the pancreas, and improves the digestion of fats. Raw, saltless sauerkraut also helps maintain the acid-alkaline balance of the body, strengthens the nerves and the immune system, and stimulates blood formation."[66]

Yields: 1 gallon

1 1/4 lb. finely chopped cabbage

3/4 lb. shredded beets

1 tablespoon wakame

1 teaspoon sea salt

Remove two leaves from the cabbage and thinly chop the rest. Mix cabbage, beet, wakame and salt in a large bowl. Use your hands to massage the cabbage to further break down the enzymes in the cabbage mixture. Transfer the mixture into glass jars, using a wooden mallet to compact leaves. Fill to the top, covering with one of the removed full leaves, and place in a cool, dark area for at least seven days.

BAKED BUTTERNUT SQUASH

Squash is a beneficial source of vitamin A, cooling and replenishing in nature, and helps resolve inflammatory conditions. Topped with walnuts and drizzled with flaxseed oil, this side dish is loaded with beneficial omega-3 fatty acids.

Serves 6-8
Cooking time: 45-60 minutes, 375 degrees

2 large butternut squash

1 teaspoon nutmeg

2 tablespoons walnuts, crushed

2 tablespoons goat cheese

Heat oven to 375 degrees. Bake squash for 45-60 minutes until tender. Slice in half, and sprinkle with nutmeg, walnuts, and goat cheese.

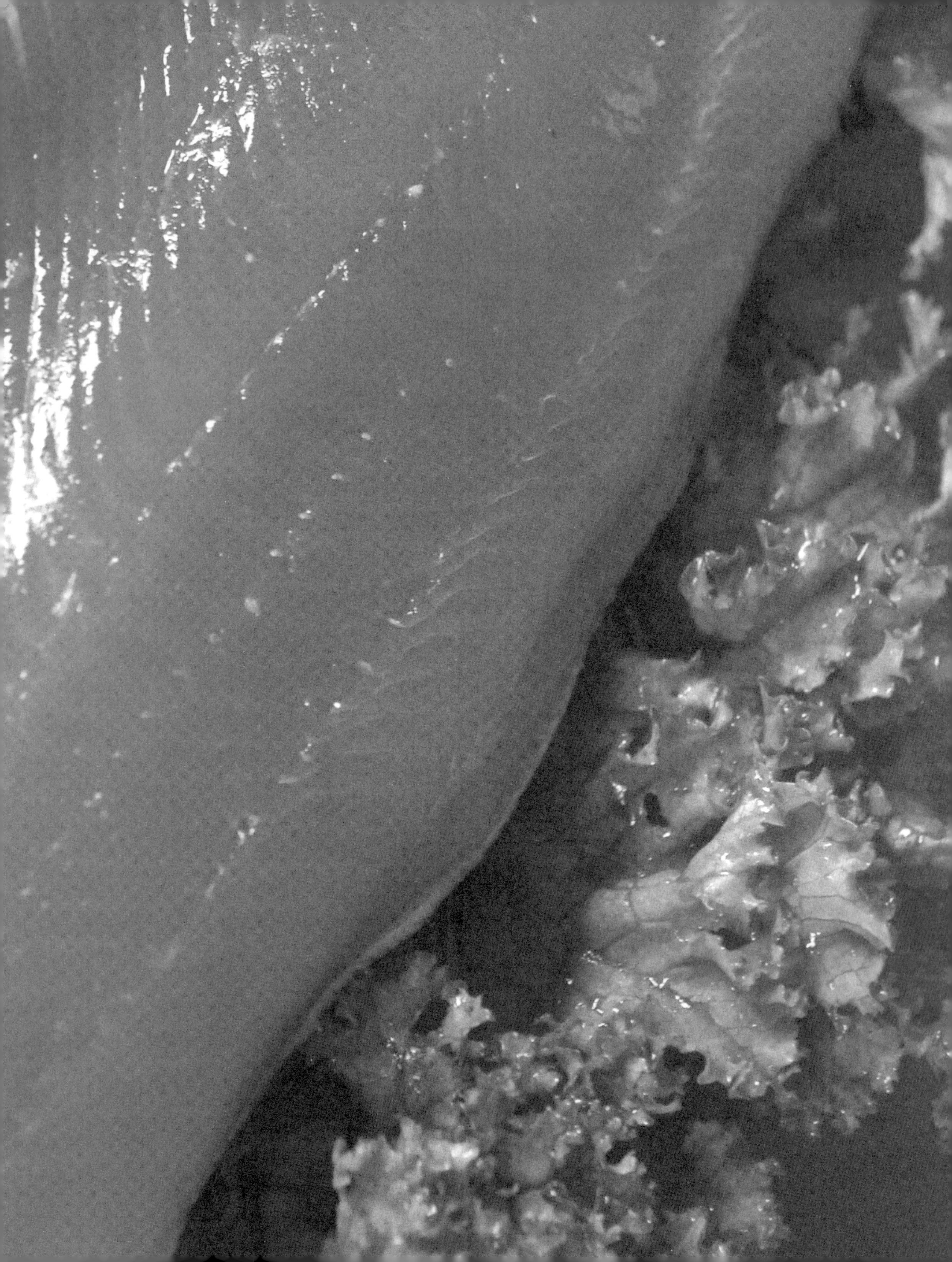

Main Attraction

When eating for fertility, your goal is to model an Asian diet. For each meal, prepare a plate filled with lightly cooked veggies, grains, and a palm-sized portion of protein, topped with your selection of "good fats and oils."

SIMPLE EATS

Using this formula, choose one item from each of the following categories to create a balanced fertile foods meal:

1. Vegetables:
Cruciferous veggies, such as cauliflower, broccoli, spinach, cabbage, bok choy, kale, collard greens, brussels sprouts, cabbage, turnip, rutabaga (these vegetables can interfere with thyroid function if eaten raw).

[Note, however, that raw seaweed, kelp, avocado, coconut, and radish can actually counter this negative effect.]

2. Grains:
Brown, black or red rice, quinoa and polenta

3. Protein:
Lentils, beans, grilled chicken, salmon, beef, tempeh or tofu

4. Good fats and oils:
Flax, pumpkin, Usana optomega oil, sesame, evening primrose, chia seed, extra virgin olive oil and or sliced avocado, goat cheese, walnuts, pinenuts, almonds, pumpkin and sesame seeds

How to cook for *The Fertile Soul?*

Broil, bake, boil, steam, grill, roast and poach

A GUIDE TO PROTEIN SOURCES

When consuming meat, always choose organic, hormone-free products. This helps avoid residual hormones and antibiotics that are used in many commercially raised animals and can disrupt your natural hormonal balance. Eating meat occasionally can increase energy and bolster energy, yin and blood. If you are experiencing PMS, hot flashes, night sweats, acne, skin irritations or have a robust constitution with a red complexion, consider limiting your consumption of red meat and opt for lighter fares such as fish and vegetarian dishes.

Beef: Use for building blood and yin fluids, strengthening bones, increasing energy, and correcting low backache and weak knees.[67] Avoid excessive consumption of red meat, because it contains arachidonic acid that can exacerbate inflammation and blood clotting.

Chicken: Use to stimulate appetite, regulate vaginal discharge, and strengthen after childbirth.[68] Chicken warms "cold conditions." including premenstrual low back pain, low libido, nighttime urination, and cold extremities.

Fish: Choose wild salmon. It is one of the richest sources of healthful omega-3 fatty acids, known to reduce blood clotting and increase circulation to damaged tissues in the body.[69] It is also essential for fetal brain development.

Vegetarian options:

Legumes and beans: "The protein from legumes can help regulate sugar, water and other aspects of metabolism, as well as promote balanced sexual activity and proper growth and development of the body."[70] Beans provide a balanced serving of protein, carbohydrates, fat, vitamins and minerals. Soak beans and legumes overnight to increase digestibility.

Tempeh: Asian tempeh is a good source of Vitamin B12. B12 is most commonly available in animal products, and in addition to omega-3 fatty acids is an essential component in the development of a healthy baby.

Tofu is a good source of B vitamins and minerals, including calcium, phosphorous, iron, sodium, and potassium.[71] It is cooling, so therefore appropriate if you have excess heat signs or desire to replenish an overstressed adrenal and reproductive system. If you lack adequate warmth, it is best enjoyed with spices such as ginger to protect digestive function.

TRI-TIP ROAST

For those experiencing exceptionally light periods or amenorrhea, grass-fed beef helps build the blood and increase energy levels.[72] Tri-tip roast is delicious served with yam casserole (On the Side) and grateful greens (Slowly with Salad). If you have PMS, clotted periods, headaches and pain at ovulation, add a side of horseradish to help move stagnant energy.

Serves 4 with leftovers
Cooking time: 40-60 minutes, 325 degrees

1 1/2 - 2 pounds grass-fed tri-tip roast

Marinade:

4 tablespoons extra virgin olive oil

2 tablespoons minced garlic

2 teaspoons dijon mustard

2 teaspoons turmeric

1 teaspoon cinnamon

Sea salt or dulse flakes to taste

In a bowl, whisk together olive oil, garlic, mustard and spices. Make slits along the meat, and rub on marinade. Seal in a plastic food storage bag from 4 hours to overnight. Preheat oven to 325 degrees, place roast in baking pan, and slow cook for 40 minutes to 1 hour, until meat reaches the desired level of doneness. Remove the roast, and let sit for approximately 10-15 minutes; it will continue to cook on the counter.

Note: Use a meat thermometer to gauge: medium rare, 145°F; medium, 160°F; well done, 170°F

BLACK BEAN BURGERS

Featured recipe in Cooking for Fertility DVD with Tiffany Pollard and Kathryn Flynn

Both black beans and lentils benefit fertility. Black beans fortify the kidneys and enhance fertility by helping to resolve low back pain and low libido, while replenishing your deepest reserves.[73] In addition, sunflower seeds introduce a healthful dose of polyunsaturated fats.[74] Serve with yam fries (On the Side) and coleslaw (Slowly with Salad).

Serves 4
Cooking time: 10 to 15 minutes

1 cup black beans (1 15-ounce can), without the juice

1 small carrot, chopped or grated

1/3 cup onion (about 1/4 of an onion)

3/4 to 1 cup crushed gluten-free crackers OR 3/4 cup wheat-free bread crumbs

2 to 3 cloves chopped garlic

1 tablespoon Herb de Provence

Sea salt to taste (I use about 1/2 teaspoon)

1 tablespoon black sesame seeds

1 egg (optional)

2 to 3 tablespoons unrefined olive oil or coconut oil

Place all ingredients in food processor and pulse until thoroughly combined. Form mixture into patties or smaller "cakes." If they are not holding together because they are too "wet," add more crackers. If they are too crumbly, add an egg. Place in an oiled skillet and cook 5 to 7 minutes on each side or until browned. Serve with pumpkin seed pesto (Snack and Appetize) on top, over some raw or steamed greens, or with sprouted grain buns.

TURKEY MEATLOAF

"Melatonin, a hormone produced by the pineal gland, is said to reduce stress, boost immunity, deepen sleep, and promote longevity."[75] In Chinese medicine, ample melatonin production is a direct reflection of your kidney and adrenal performance, the paired organs of the reproductive system. Turkey contains tryptophan, the precursor needed for creating melatonin. By eating foods with tryptophan and B vitamins, you can reduce the impact of stress on your body and replenish all aspects of your vitality. (Remember, don't supplement with melatonin directly; eat food containing its precursors.)

Yields: 1 medium loaf
Cooking time: 55-60 minutes, 375 degrees

1 cup finely minced broccoli and cauliflower

1 clove garlic, minced

1 medium onion, minced

1 pound organic ground turkey

2 eggs or egg replacement (basic ingredients)

1 cup wheat-free bread crumbs

1 tbsp wheat-free tamari

1 teaspoon Herb de Provence

1/2 cup of marinara sauce plus 1 tablespoon

1 teaspoon extra virgin olive oil

Preheat oven to 375. Place vegetables, garlic and onion in a food processor and blend thoroughly. Combine meat and eggs. Add processed vegetables, breadcrumbs, seasonings, 1 tablespoon of marinara and olive oil, mixing until thoroughly combined. Place in loaf pan and top with remaining marinara sauce.

ROAST CHICKEN WITH STUFFING

Chicken supports digestion by increasing the flow of qi in the body.[76] Eat soups with a chicken base on a cool winter evening to warm you from the inside out and to resolve cold conditions, including premenstrual low back pain, low libido, and nighttime urination. Serve with Quinoa Tabouli and Cruciferous Crunch (On the Side).

Serves 4-6 with leftovers
Cooking time: 45-60 minutes, 350 degrees

Whole organic chicken (approximately 4 pounds)

1 tablespoon extra virgin olive oil

1 teaspoon Herb de Provence

1 teaspoon lemon thyme seasoning

Salt and Pepper to taste

Stuffing

3 cups of wheat-free bread crumbs, 2 inch pieces

1/4 onion, finely chopped

1/4 cup celery, finely chopped

1/2 teaspoon fresh sage

1/2 teaspoon fresh thyme

1/8 cup goji berries

1/8 cup slivered almonds

1 tablespoon extra virgin olive oil

2 tablespoons chicken or vegetable broth

Preheat oven to 350 degrees. Rub chicken with olive oil and seasonings. For stuffing, mix all ingredients together and place inside chicken breast. Place chicken breast in roasting dish with shallow layer of water. Bake 45-60 minutes. Use leftovers for soup or add to spaghetti sauce.

POACHED SALMON WITH PINEAPPLE SAUCE

Featured recipe in Cooking for Fertility DVD with Tiffany Pollard and Kathryn Flynn

Wild salmon is one of the richest sources of healthful omega-3 fatty acids, known to reduce blood clotting and increase circulation to damaged tissues in the body.[77] It is also an essential component for in-utero brain development of babies. In this recipe, we have added implantation-enhancing bromelain in pineapple. Enjoy salmon several times a week.

Serves 3 to 4
Cooking time: 10 to 12 minutes

4 cups of organic chicken or veggie broth

1 pound wild salmon fillets

Salt and pepper to taste

Chopped parsley and or red bell pepper for garnish

Optional: 4 pineapple slices set on side of each plate

Pineapple sauce

Yields: 3/4 cup

1/2 cup fresh or frozen pineapple, chopped

2 to 3 Tablespoons agave nectar

2 tablespoons Dijon mustard

Fill a skillet one-third full of broth and put on medium low heat; add salmon and cover (you want for the liquid to be at least half way up on the side of the highest part of the fish fillet). Turn the heat low, so salmon poaches in the broth and steam, until bright pink and easily flaked with a knife (approximately 10-12 minutes). In a blender or food processor, combine pineapple, agave, and mustard. Plate the fish and drizzle with pineapple sauce.

SALMON CAKES

In TCM, the rich pink color of salmon indicates it has a warming effect, helpful in resolving premenstrual low back pain, low libido, and nighttime urination and general cold feelings. Apart from its omega-3 fatty acid benefits, salmon is a significant source of calcium.[78]

Serves 4-6
Cooking time: 5-10 minutes

1/2 medium red onion

1 clove garlic, crushed

1 pound salmon fillet, cooked

2 teaspoons fresh rosemary

1 cup wheat-free bread crumbs

1 egg or egg replacer (basic ingredients)

1 tablespoon extra virgin olive oil

Place onion and garlic in food processor and pulse until finely shredded. Add salmon, rosemary, bread crumbs and egg, pulsing until thoroughly combined. Form patties or balls. Lightly pan fry with olive oil over medium heat, three minutes on each side.

GARLIC CASHEW CHICKEN

Chicken supports digestion by increasing the flow of qi in the body.[79] Cashews are an abundant source of magnesium, necessary for calcium and vitamin D absorption as well as the relaxation response. Other magnesium-rich foods are seaweeds, aduki and black beans, barley and rice.[80] To enhance the peace and serenity of this dish, serve over brown rice at a candlelit table.

Serves 4
Cooking time: 15-20 minutes

1 cup cashews

1 tablespoon olive oil

1 1/2 cups diced chicken

1/2 cup onions

1 1/2 cups peppers (red and green)

1/4 cup of goji berries

Marinade

1 tablespoon olive oil

2 tablespoons sesame oil

2 teaspoons wheat-free tamari

2 teaspoons minced garlic

1 teaspoon minced ginger

Blend olive oil, sesame oil, tamari, garlic, and ginger and marinade chicken. Stir fry cashews in 1 tablespoon of olive oil for 2-3 minutes on medium-high heat, then set aside. Add marinated chicken to pan and stir-fry for 5 minutes before adding onions and peppers. Continue to cook for an additional 5-8 minutes or until onions are translucent. Add cashews and gojis in final moments to warm, and serve on brown rice.

PAD THAI

Traditional pad Thai is made with peanuts, but we prefer almonds, used in the Ayurvedic tradition to bolster spirituality and improve reproductive function.[81] Almonds are also an excellent source of protein and contain zinc and Vitamin E, which support the health of the uterine lining and placenta in pregnancy. Almond skins are also a great source of calcium.

Serves 4-6
Cooking time: 15-20 minutes

8 ounces linguine noodles (spelt, brown rice or quinoa)

1/2 cup organic unsalted almonds, crushed

3 tablespoons wheat-free tamari

2 tablespoons lemon juice

3 tablespoons water

Rice vinegar

1 tablespoon extra virgin olive oil

2 cloves garlic, chopped

1/2 cup onion, chopped

1 cup snow peas

3 cups fresh bean sprouts

1/3 cup green onions, thinly sliced

Cook noodles, and drain. Blend almonds in food processor. Combine tamari, lemon juice, water and rice vinegar. Heat oil in skillet, adding garlic and onions. Slowly add snow peas and bean sprouts. When tender, add noodles, almonds, and green onions, then slowly pour liquid mixture over top and serve.

BROWN RICE PIZZA

Here is a delicious variation on traditional pizza with the added nourishment of brown rice, containing more than 70 antioxidants. Enjoy with or without cheese alternative. See topping varieties below.

Yields one medium sized pizza
Cooking time: 20-25 minutes, 450 degrees

3 cups cooked brown rice, warm

1/2 cup onions, finely chopped

2 tablespoons extra virgin olive oil

1 teaspoon Italian seasoning

Preheat oven to 450 degrees. Pulse all ingredients in a food processor, and press onto a lightly greased pizza pan. Bake until golden brown. Add desired toppings and bake until cheese melts.

Suggested toppings:

Simple: marinara (spaghetti squash with marinara), basil, and goat cheese

California Style: pumpkin pesto sauce (pesto spirals), leftover salmon, olives, red onion, capers, and goat cheese

The Works: 1/2 pumpkin pesto, 1/2 marinara, with leftover chicken, bell peppers, onions, yams, mushrooms, and almond cheese

STUFFED PORTOBELLO MUSHROOMS

This dish bolsters immunity with mushrooms, builds blood with spinach, offers omega-3 fatty acids in walnuts, and adds a serving of full-fat dairy with goat cheese. Serve with Moroccan tabouli (on the side).

Serves 2-4
Cooking time: 8-10 minutes, 375 degrees

1 tablespoon + 1 tablespoon extra virgin olive oil

2 cloves garlic, minced

12 ounces fresh spinach

1 cup tomatoes, chopped

4 large portobello mushrooms

1/3 cup goat cheese

1/8 cup walnuts, crushed

Sea salt or dulse flakes to taste

Preheat oven to 375 degrees. Heat 1 tablespoon olive oil in a skillet, and add garlic and spinach, stirring until wilted. Remove, and add tomatoes.

Scoop out insides from mushroom caps, rinse and dry thoroughly. Brush mushrooms with 1 tablespoon olive oil and spoon spinach mixture into caps. Sprinkle goat cheese on top and top with walnuts, if desired, and bake on a cookie sheet for 8-10 minutes.

SEAFOOD DINNER

Both oysters and clams can build reproductive essence. Oysters, commonly considered an aphrodisiac, help build blood and yin and often are used to overcome nervous conditions and indecision. Clams help regulate vaginal discharge, edema, and excess vaginal bleeding.[82] Favor oysters if you have cold symptoms, such as premenstrual low back pain, low libido, nighttime urination, or are generally cold in nature. Eating clams helps if you have hot symptoms, such as short cycles, scant cervical mucus, night sweats, hot flashes, or back or knee weakness.

Serves 5-6
Cooking time: 5-10 minutes

1 pound clams or oysters

1/4 cup roasted pumpkin seeds, crushed

1/4 cup almond flour

2 eggs, beaten

1 tablespoon extra virgin olive oil

Rinse and drain clams or oysters; dry on paper towels. Combine pumpkin seeds with almond flour. Beat eggs with a fork. Dip seafood in eggs, then in almond meal mixture. Heat olive oil in skillet, and sauté seafood. Serve with choice of vegetable sides.

TILAPIA WITH SAUTÉED SPINACH

Spinach is rich in iron and chlorophyll, helping build and enrich blood. If you have short cycles, scant cervical mucus, night sweats, hot flashes, and back or knee weakness, favor white fish like tilapia to cool your heat.

Serves 2
Cooking time: 15 minutes, 400 degrees

1/2 cup onion, minced

6 ounces fresh spinach

1 teaspoon turmeric

1 teaspoon extra virgin olive oil

2 fillets tilapia

1 teaspoon wheat-free tamari

Sauté onion, spinach and turmeric in olive oil, until liquid evaporates. Set aside. Rinse fish fillets, and place on platter. Sprinkle with tamari sauce, and top with a thin layer of spinach mixture. Roll each filet, and secure with two toothpicks. Bake in a glass dish at 400 degrees for 15 minutes. Garnish with lemon slices.

EGGPLANT PARMESAN CASSEROLE

Eggplant, a rich source of bioflavonoids, is an ideal treatment for stagnant blood in the uterus. On an emotional level, it is believed to help resolve repressed emotion affecting both the uterus and liver. Due to eggplant's hemostatic qualities, do not consume large amounts during pregnancy.[83]

Serves 4-6

Cooking time: 40 minutes + 50 minutes, 350 degrees

1 large eggplant, sliced 1/2-inch thick

2 eggs

2 tablespoons almond, hemp, or goat milk

2 cups wheat-free bread crumbs

3/4 cup goat cheese

2 cups marinara sauce

Salt and ground pepper, as desired

1 teaspoon extra virgin olive oil (for glass plan)

1 tablespoon pine nuts to top (optional)

Preheat oven to 350 degrees. If making from scratch, prepare marinara sauce (see spaghetti squash with marinara recipe later in this section). In a medium to large bowl, whisk eggs and milk alternative. Place bread crumbs in a separate bowl. Dip each slice of eggplant in egg mixture, then crumbs, placing on greased baking sheet. Bake for 40 minutes, or until crumbs are browned, flipping once. Remove from oven. Create two layers of the following in a medium glass plan: marinara sauce, eggplant slices, goat cheese and pine nuts if desired. Bake for 50 minutes or until tender.

YAM AND BLACK BEAN FAJITAS

In TCM, black beans are used to fortify the kidneys and enhance fertility.[84] Yams are a sweet source of vitamin A source, and large amounts should be avoided if you have PCOS or insulin resistance. Pumpkin seeds have high levels of zinc and omega fatty acids, while kale abounds with blood-building chlorophyll and iron.

Serves 4-6
Cooking time: 15 minutes, 325 degrees

1 package corn tortillas

1 tablespoon extra virgin olive oil

1 teaspoon fajita spice

1/4 cup water

1/2 cup chopped onion

1 clove garlic, minced

1/2 cup red peppers

1 cup kale, minced

1 large yam, cooked and cubed

1 cup black beans, cooked and pureed (see cooking beans and legumes – On the Side)

1/2 cup goat cheese, crumbled

1/4 cup pumpkin seeds

Over medium heat, sauté olive oil, fajita spice, water, onion, garlic, red peppers, and kale until tender. At the same time, heat corn tortillas in the oven at 325 degrees until warm. Serve buffet style with yams and black beans, guacamole and salsa (On the Side), goat cheese, and pumpkin seeds.

PESTO SPIRALS

Basil is one of the primary spices used to calm the mind.[85] It will help you if you suffer from premenstrual symptoms, irritability, headaches, or have breast tenderness at ovulation. Pumpkin seeds are loaded with omega-3 fatty acids and zinc. They help resolve impotence and fortify sperm reservoirs.[86]

Serves 2-4
Cooking time: 15-20 minutes

12 ounce package brown rice, quinoa or spelt rotini, cooked

2 links organic sausage, cooked and thinly sliced

Pesto Sauce:

Featured recipe in Cooking for Fertility DVD with Tiffany Pollard and Kathryn Flynn

Yields: 1 1/2 cups

2 cups packed fresh basil (or 1 cup basil and 1 cup kale de-stemmed)

3/4 cup pumpkin seeds

1/2 cup extra virgin olive oil

3 garlic cloves chopped

2 tablespoons balsamic vinegar

Salt and pepper to taste

Optional: reduce olive oil by 1/4 cup and add 1/2 ripe avocado for creamy texture

Begin by chopping basil and kale in food processor, then add pumpkin seeds and garlic, continuing to blend. Slowly add olive oil, forming a thick, smooth paste. Add balsamic vinegar and desired seasoning. Serve over wheat-free pasta, cooked according to package directions, with sausage. Save extra pesto sauce for pizza.

SPAGHETTI SQUASH WITH CHICKEN MARINARA

Spaghetti squash is a wonderful alternative to traditional pastas. Squash is a good source of Vitamin A and is cooling and replenishing for overstressed adrenal and reproductive systems.[87] It is delicious paired with chicken marinara, a truly heart-warming sauce.

Serves 4-6
Cooking time: 45-50 minutes, 400 degrees

1 large spaghetti squash

1 teaspoon extra virgin olive oil

2 cups marinara sauce

Prepare marinara sauce on next page. While it is simmering, bake whole squash at 400 degrees for 45 minutes, until soft. Slice in half, and remove and discard seeds. Scoop spaghetti from the squash with a fork and sauté over medium heat for 2 minutes with olive oil. Top with chicken marinara sauce and enjoy!

Marinara

Yields: 12 cups
Cooking time: 2 hours

3-4 tablespoons olive oil

2 cloves garlic, minced

1 onion, chopped

9 tomatoes, chopped

1 green pepper, chopped

1 red pepper, chopped

10 mushrooms, chopped

2 large cans diced tomatoes

2 8-ounce cans tomato paste

2 teaspoons basil

1 teaspoon rosemary

1 teaspoon oregano

1 teaspoon parsley

1 cup rotisserie chicken (optional)

Salt and pepper to taste

In a large pot, heat oil; add garlic and onions, and sauté until soft. Add the other fresh and canned vegetables, along with the tomato paste. Let simmer on low heat uncovered, adding spices to taste. Leave on low heat for 2 hours or longer, adding pieces of roasted chicken, if desired. Serve over spaghetti squash or try brown rice, spelt or quinoa pasta.

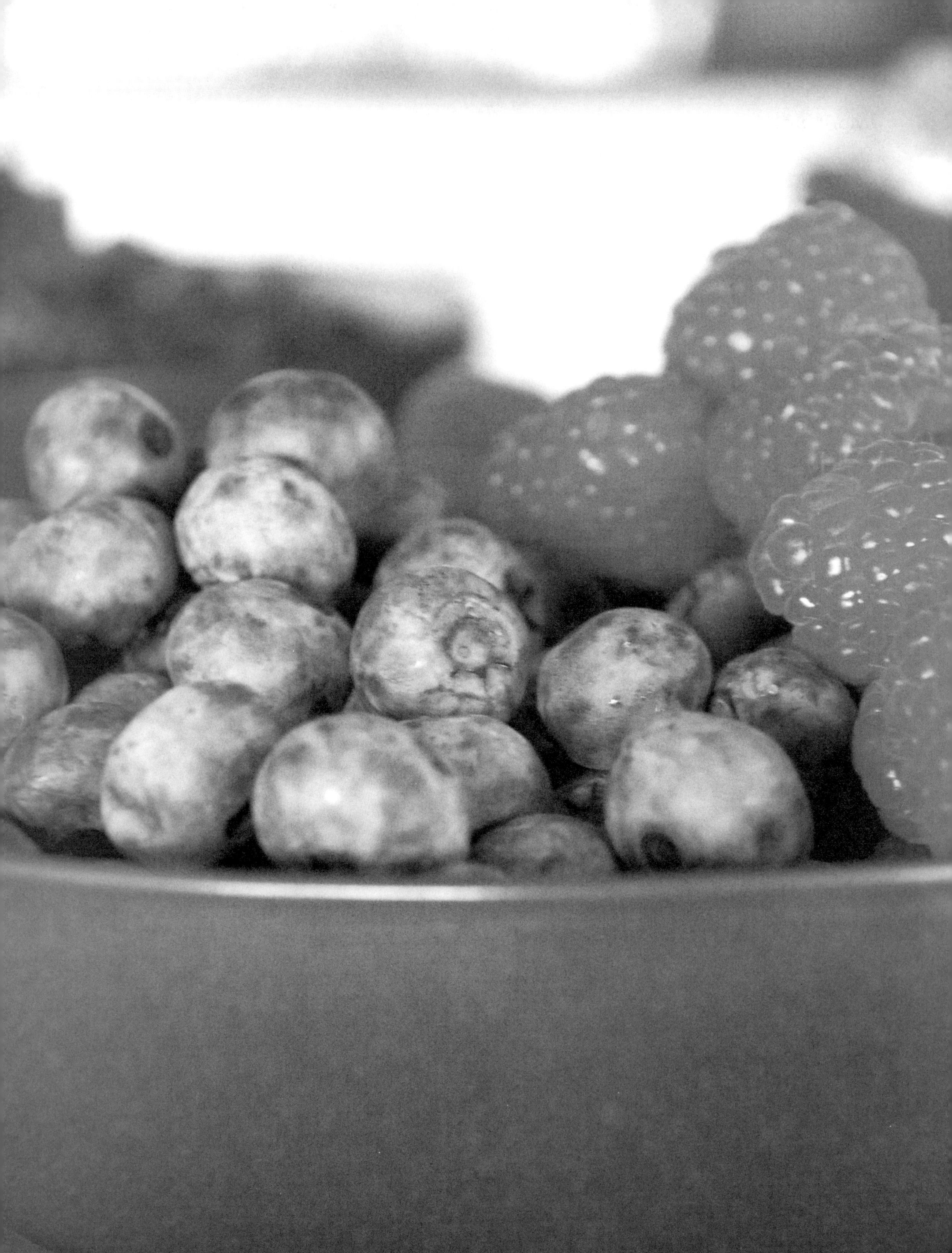

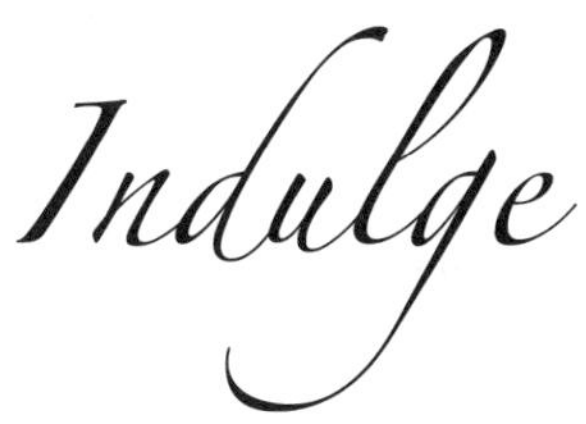

We wholeheartedly believe that it is important to treat yourself. In fact, we recommend that you follow the fertility guidelines 80 per cent of the time and indulge wisely the other 20 per cent. The one rule we adamantly require, however, is that indulgence be guilt-free.

Tips for smart fertility indulgences:

- Use natural sugar sources, such as fruit (see Appetize and Snack section for healing benefits), and favor low-glycemic agave nectar as a sweetener to help keep blood sugar levels stable and avoid fluctuating hormone and energy levels.
- Eat fruits in their whole form, not as juice. Juices are loaded with sugar, producing dampness and encouraging yeast formation in the body. Unsweetened juices lack the fiber that helps slow absorption of natural sugar from whole fruits.
- Avoid foods sweetened with sugar, corn syrup, or artificial sweeteners. Commercially prepared baked goods, pastries and sodas are generally full of white flour, sugars, or chemicals that disrupt your body's natural processes. Let your body adjust to the way it was supposed to eat, focusing on whole foods that come from the earth.
- Eat dark chocolate to get the benefits of flavonoids to encourage blood flow and arginine to improve egg quality. Be sure to choose varieties that are at least 70 per cent cacao or more.
- Favor lower-glycemic sweeteners to help keep blood-sugar levels stable and avoid fluctuating hormone and energy levels.

  In these recipes we have chosen to use agave nectar, and it is important to note that not all agave nectars are created equally. Be sure to look for raw, organic, blue agave nectar sources. Please note that although agave nectar metabolizes more slowly in the system, it is still a sweetener and therefore impacts blood-sugar levels. All sugars, even those that are natural, should only be used in moderation.

Sweetener	Replace 1 cup of refined sugar with:
Agave nectar	¾ cup
Brown rice syrup	1 cup
Blackstrap molasses	½ cup
Raw honey	¾ cup
Maple syrup	¾ cup
Xylitol	1 cup

BANANA WALNUT BREAD

Bananas help nourish an overstressed system and yin fluids. Avoid bananas if you are prone to dampness or excess yeast. Walnuts add a healthy dose of omega-3 fatty acids, and the protein balances the carbohydrates.

Yields medium loaf
Cooking time: 45 minutes, 325 degrees

2 cups walnuts, finely chopped

3 bananas, mashed

2 tablespoons ghee (Basic Ingredients)

2 eggs or egg alternative (Basic Ingredients)

1 tablespoon agave nectar

1 teaspoon vanilla

1 teaspoon baking soda

1 teaspoon cinnamon

Preheat oven to 325 degrees. In a food processor, finely chop 2 cups walnuts. Beat together mashed banana, ghee, eggs, agave and vanilla. Fold in walnut mixture, baking soda and cinnamon and mix until smooth. Spoon mixture into lightly greased loaf pan, and bake for 45 minutes or until inserted toothpick comes out clean.

BERRY COBBLER

This sweet treat supports the free flow of blood and energy between the heart and the uterus. Blueberries nourish kidney yin, supporting the resolution of "urinary, sexual and reproductive imbalances."[88] Fresh raspberries "enrich and cleanse the blood of toxins" and "regulate the menstrual cycle."[89] Oats add substance to the diet, calming the nervous system and inviting the relaxation response, so important for fertility. Flaxseed with its omega-3 fatty acids helps resolve blood stagnations like clotting.

Serves 4-6
Cooking time: 45 minutes, 375 degrees

4 cups fresh blueberries or raspberries

1/4 cup agave nectar

Juice of 1/2 fresh lemon

2 tablespoons brown rice flour

Topping:

3/4 cup almond flour

3/4 cup rolled oats

2 tablespoons ground flaxseed

1 teaspoon baking powder

1/2 cup melted clarified butter/ghee

1/3 cup agave nectar

Preheat oven to 375 degrees. Combine berries, agave, lemon juice and brown rice flour. In a separate bowl combine dry topping ingredients, and knead butter and agave nectar into dry mixture. Place fruit in lightly greased baking dish, and cover with topping. Bake for 45 minutes or until golden brown.

FERTILE SOUL COOKIES

The sweet healing properties of these cookies help soothe symptoms of PMS. Oats calm the heart, while coconut nourishes yin fluids like semen and cervical mucus.

Yields: 12-15 cookies
Cooking time: 15 minutes, 350 degrees

1 cup brown rice flour

1/2 cup tapioca flour

3/4 cup rolled oats

1/2 cup shredded unsweetened coconut

1/2 teaspoon xantham gum

1/4 cup melted clarified butter/ghee

1 teaspoon vanilla

1/2 cup agave nectar

1/4 cup dark chocolate chips

1/4 cup pumpkin seeds, crushed

1/8 cup goji berries

Preheat oven to 350 degrees. Combine flours and oats, coconut and xantham in a bowl. Next add melted butter, vanilla and agave nectar mixing until thoroughly combined. Finally add chocolate chips, pumpkin seeds and goji berries and chill in the refrigerator about one hour. Drop spoonfuls of dough unto lightly greased cookie sheets. Bake for 15 minutes, remove from oven, and leave on pan for an additional 5 minutes.

GRILLED MANGO

Mango builds kidney yin fluids and replenishes overstressed adrenal and reproductive systems. Served with goat milk, this dessert nourishes your deepest reserves of yin and blood, cooling excess heat or symptoms like night sweats, hot flashes, and hot skin rashes.

Serves 2-4
Cooking time: 5-10 minutes

2 mangoes, peeled, pitted and sliced

3 tablespoons fresh raspberries to garnish

1 tablespoon slivered almonds

1/2 cup Goat yogurt (optional)

Preheat grill. Grill mango slices over medium heat until warmed through, about 3 minutes per side, flipping once. Remove from heat, and cover with a dollop of goat yogurt and fresh raspberries with slivered almonds to top. Serve immediately.

CRISPY TREATS

In this dessert, the sugar in the chocolate is stabilized by the protein and fat in the nuts. When eaten in moderation, this supports the movement of qi and blood. The flavonoids in dark chocolate increase blood flow and ease inflammation.

Yields: 16 bars
Cooking time: 5-10 minutes

1 cup almond butter

1/4 cup dark chocolate chips

1 teaspoon vanilla

1/4 cup agave nectar

3 cups brown rice crisp cereal

1/4 cup coconut

1 teaspoon cinnamon

In a pot, heat almond butter, chocolate chips, vanilla and agave nectar over low heat, until smooth. Take off stove, and mix in cereal, coconut and cinnamon. Smooth into flat pan, refrigerate for at least two hours and cut into bars.

SWEET POTATO PIE

Sweet potatoes have yin building properties to help you rebuild your essence and reconnect with your roots. They are also high in Vitamin A for enhanced vision. This pie can also be prepared with yams.

Yields: 1 medium sized pie
Cooking time: 30-40 minutes, 375 degrees

1 1/2 cups sweet potatoes, cooked, peeled and pureed (approximately 4)

1/2 cup agave nectar

3 tablespoons molasses

1/2 cup almond, hemp, rice or goat milk

1/2 teaspoon vanilla

1 teaspoon cinnamon

1 teaspoon ground ginger

1/4 teaspoon ground cloves

Combine sweet potato puree with agave nectar, molasses and milk alternative. Fold in vanilla and spices. Pour into muffin tins or a wheat or gluten-free pie shell and bake at 375 degrees for 30-40 minutes.

COCONUT RICE PUDDING

Slowly simmered, this dessert supports all organs classified under the water element in TCM: reproductive, adrenal system, and kidneys. Coconut and cinnamon optimize digestion.

Serves 2-4
Cooking time: 30 minutes

1 cup brown rice, cooked

1 cup coconut milk

1 cup almond, hemp, rice or goat milk

1 cup water

1 tablespoon agave nectar

1/4 teaspoon cinnamon

1/2 teaspoon vanilla

1 tablespoon toasted walnuts or almonds

1/2 tablespoon goji berries

1 tablespoon pumpkin seeds, crushed (optional)

Combine rice, milks, water, and agave in saucepan. Bring to a boil, and reduce heat. Simmer for 20 minutes, stirring occasionally. Remove from heat; add cinnamon and vanilla. Top with toasted nuts, goji berries and seeds as desired.

CHOCOLATE COVERED STRAWBERRIES

Dark chocolate is a friendly monounsaturated fat that has some strong implications for fertility. Research shows that simply the smell of chocolate can increase theta waves, which promote the relaxation response. Also chocolate contain flavonoids, known to help elevate mood, promote blood flow, ease inflammation, and inhibit the formation of blood clots. Chocolate also contains arginine, which specifically increases blood flow to the uterus and ovaries. Avoid chocolate and supplements containing L-arginine if you experience heat signs, particularly with skin eruptions like herpes.

Yields: 12-15 pieces
Cooking time: 5-10 minutes

12 - 15 strawberries

1 cup dark chocolate chips

In a double boiler slowly melt dark chocolate. Dip washed and dried berries in chocolate, and place on baking sheet lined with parchment paper. Refrigerate for 15-20 minutes and serve.

CHOCOLATE MOUSSE

Featured recipe in Cooking for Fertility DVD with Tiffany Pollard and Kathryn Flynn

Tofu provides a healthy yin-nourishing alternative to traditional heavy cream and raw-egg mousses. The hint of cinnamon in this dark chocolate decadence sparks sensual and digestive energies.

Serves 4 to 6
Cooking time: 5-10 minutes

1 package Silken tofu

2 to 4 tablespoons agave syrup

2 teaspoon vanilla extract

10 ounces dark chocolate, melted

1/2 teaspoon cinnamon (optional)

1/2 avocado (optional)

In a blender or food processor, puree tofu and optional avocado, with agave, vanilla and optional cinnamon until perfectly smooth. Add melted chocolate and mix until fully combined. Pour mixture in a bowl, and let sit in the fridge for at least 4 hours.

RANDINE'S POPCORN

An all-time favorite for movie time at the Fertile Soul, sweetened with agave and almond butter to stabilize energy and blood sugar levels.

Yields: 8 cups
Cooking time: 10 minutes

3 tablespoons ghee (see Basic Ingredients)

1/3 cup popcorn kernels

Salt to taste

Topping

1/4 cup ghee/clarified butter

1/2 cup agave nectar (or up to 1/4 cup maple butter)

1/2 cup almond butter

Heat the ghee in a saucepan on high heat. Test it by adding a few kernels. When they pop, add the rest. Cover and shake the pan slightly while the corn pops, leaving the cover ajar so steam is released. At the same time add the topping ingredients to a separate pan and melt over medium heat. Once the popping stops, remove pan from heat, put popcorn in serving dish and add topping.

Lifestyle Recommendations

Meditate: Sit quietly and allow thoughts to pass through the mind without attaching.

Trust yourself: Develop self-confidence; learn to listen to inner voice and say No without a reason or excuse. Adopt self-expression affirmations: "I feel," "I feel like," "I like my."

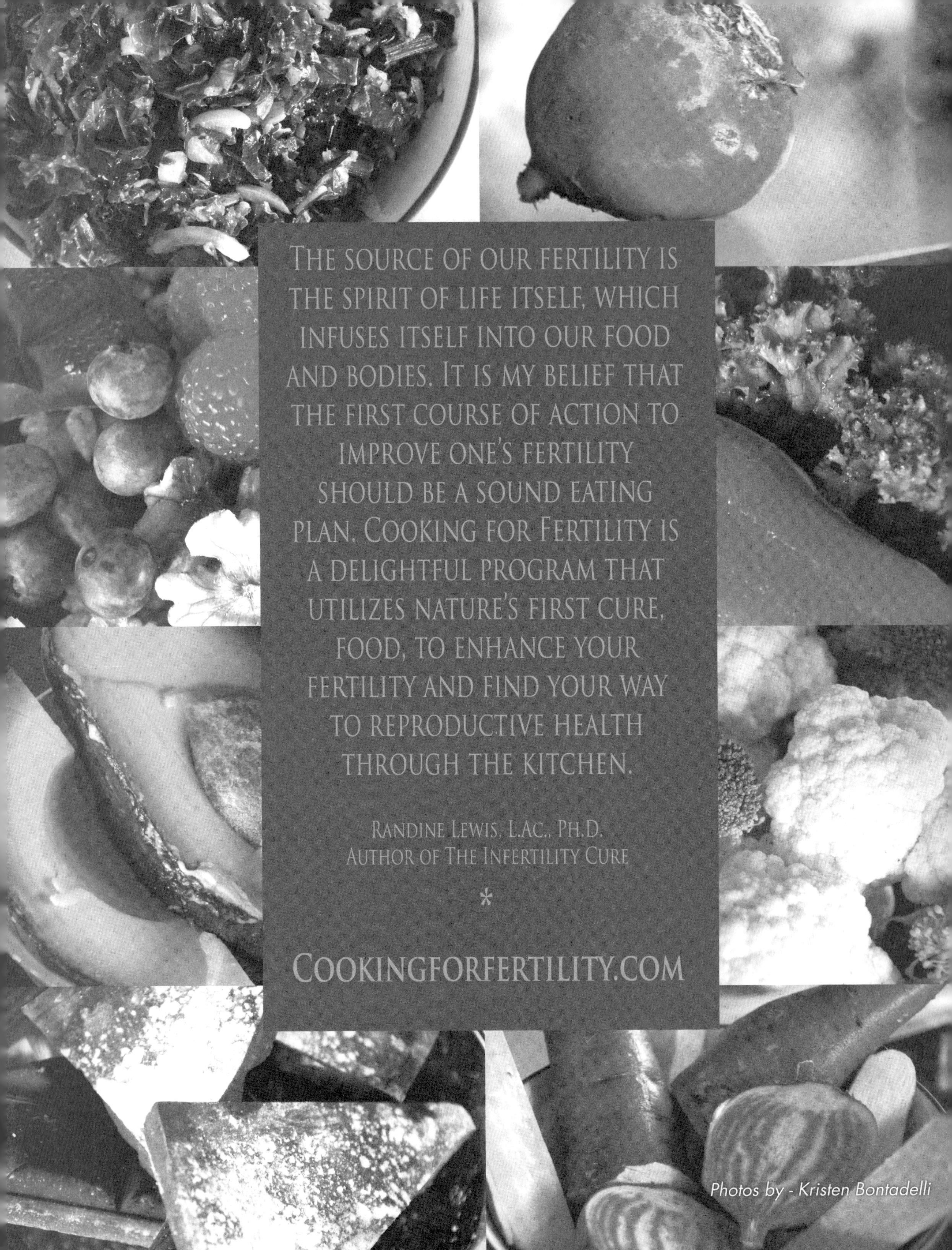
THE SOURCE OF OUR FERTILITY IS THE SPIRIT OF LIFE ITSELF, WHICH INFUSES ITSELF INTO OUR FOOD AND BODIES. IT IS MY BELIEF THAT THE FIRST COURSE OF ACTION TO IMPROVE ONE'S FERTILITY SHOULD BE A SOUND EATING PLAN. COOKING FOR FERTILITY IS A DELIGHTFUL PROGRAM THAT UTILIZES NATURE'S FIRST CURE, FOOD, TO ENHANCE YOUR FERTILITY AND FIND YOUR WAY TO REPRODUCTIVE HEALTH THROUGH THE KITCHEN.
RANDINE LEWIS, L.AC., PH.D.
AUTHOR OF THE INFERTILITY CURE
*
COOKINGFORFERTILITY.COM
Photos by - Kristen Bontadelli

Eating According to Your Symptoms and Diagnosis: Lifestyle Recommendations & Meal Plans

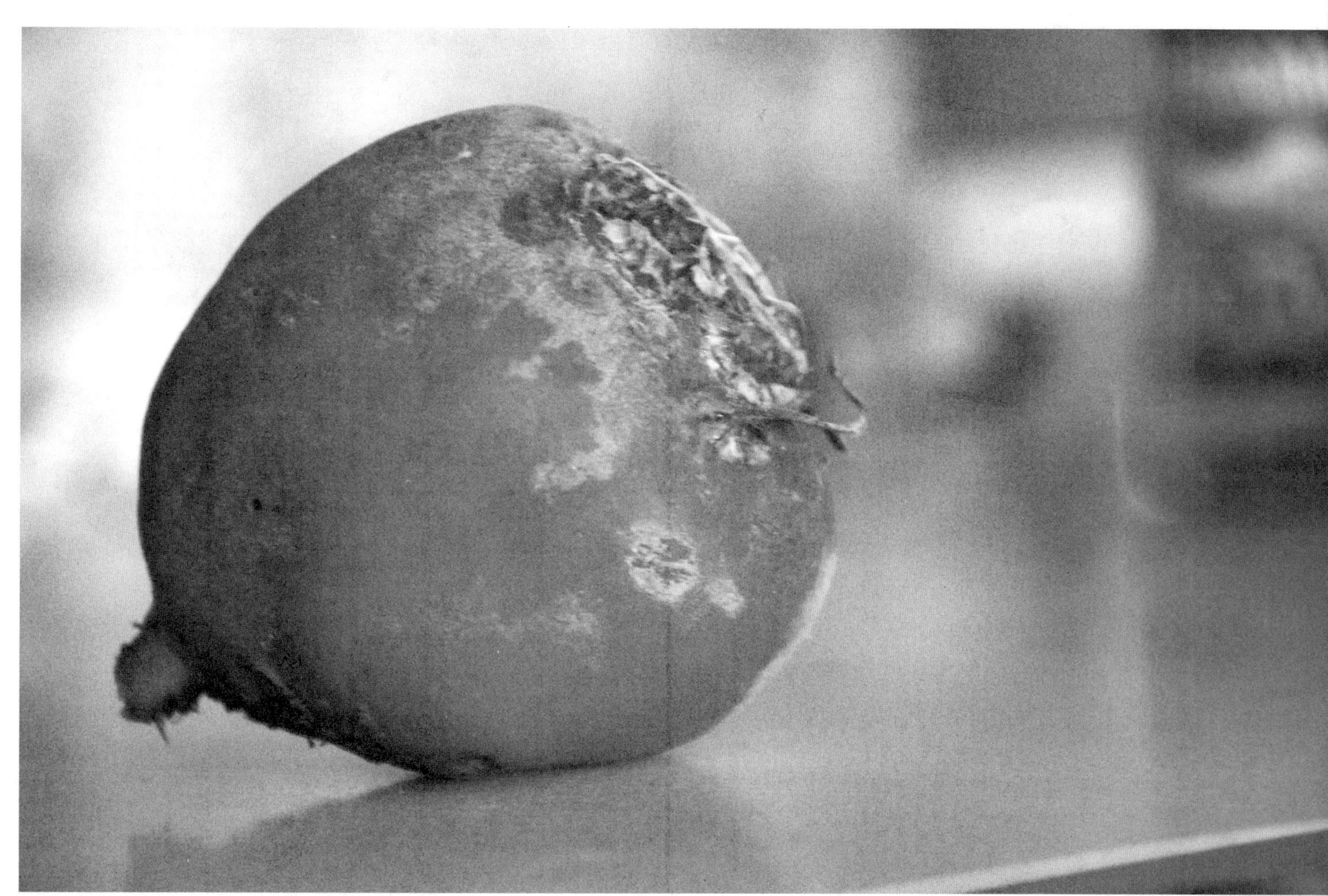

SPLEEN QI DEFICIENCY AND DAMPNESS

Spleen qi deficiency: low energy, sluggish after meals, craves sweets, loose stools, worry, spotting before menstruation, bruises easily

Dampness: pustular acne, mucus in menstrual blood, yeast infections, joint pain

Western conditions: autoimmune disorders, thyroid imbalance, obesity, candida, PCOS

Spleen health depends upon our ability to stay grounded and calm. The associated emotion of the Spleen is worry. Excessive use of the mind in thinking, studying, concentrating and memorizing over a long period of time tends to weaken the Spleen. The Chinese believe "over-thinking" or "ruminating" can inhibit the energetic processes of the Spleen. Open consideration is the most fertile ground for the Spleen energies, allowing thoughts to pass through freely, creating intention with action or releasing the thought and moving on. This frees up the Spleen energies to properly digest, transform and distribute nourishment and vital energy to all organs.

Environment: Favor dry environments and change out of wet clothes immediately

Self-nurture: Do at least one thing each day to take care of your own needs.

Journal: Write down lingering thoughts that have not produced action at the end of each day. By putting them on paper, you can release and start fresh in the morning.

Exercise: Set up a daily movement routine, using cardiovascular and muscle strength to encourage fresh blood supply and oxygen to organs, increase metabolism, lose excess weight, and resolve candida. Most importantly: clear your mind.

Yoga: Wind Removing Posture: lying on your back, lift up your right knee and pull it into your chest. Repeat on left leg working both the ascending and descending colon sequentially. Be sure to breathe as you optimize the processes of assimilation, digestion and release.

Qi Gong: Practice "gathering the earth" in nature to connect with the earth barefoot. Stand with your feet hip-width apart. Bend your knees slightly and pretend you are gathering leaves from the earth. Lift the leaves toward your belly and then overhead as though you are sending them into the air, making a circle with your arms and bringing them to the side. Repeat this exercise, focusing on your breath inhaling as you lift the harvest from the earth, drawing it into your center, and release it to the heavens.

Sleep: Aim to be in bed by 11pm each night and get 7-8 hours of rest to replenish your deepest reserves. Consider eating breakfast within an hour of waking, ideally between the hours of 7-9 am and 9-11 am, the corresponding times of the digestive organs: the spleen-pancreas and stomach.

Spleen Qi Deficiency Meal Plan

Foods to build energy: Barley, beef, cherries, chicken, coconut, dates, eel, figs, ginseng, goose, grapes, ham, herring, Job's tears, lentils, licorice, mackerel, microalgae, molasses, oats, octopus, potatoes, pumpkin, pumpkin seeds, rabbit, rice, royal jelly, sweet potatoes, shiitake mushroom, squash, sturgeon, tofu, yams

Sunday	Monday	Tuesday	Wednesday	Thursday	Friday	Saturday
Breakfast						
Root hash trio	Gourmet oatmeal	Quinoa "Mother of Grains"	Sprouted fertility loaf with almond butter	Cocoberry pancakes	Quinoa "Mother of Grains"	Tofu scramble
Snack						
Blueberry smoothie	Rice bread with nut butter	Pear with nut butter	Pumpkin seeds and goji berries	Half serving of gourmet oatmeal	Sprouted loaf with nut butter	Cranberries and walnuts
Lunch						
White bean stew Brown rice	Quinoa tabouli Mighty greens Black beans	Fertility stew	Lentil soup Broccoli Quinoa	Black bean burger Mighty greens	Curried root stew	Black beans Avocado Brown rice Greens
Snack						
Turkey meatballs with pineapple sauce	Rice crackers Hummus	Corn tortillas Guacamole	Roasted garlic brie with crackers	Pear with nut butter	Turkey, avocado and kale wraps with hummus	Ginger sesame asparagus spears
Dinner						
Tri-tip Loaded yams	Brown rice pasta Pumpkin pesto	Black bean and yam fajitas	Spaghetti squash Chicken marinara	Poached salmon Cruciferous crunch Moroccan pilaf	Tri-tip Loaded yams Mighty greens	Stuffed portobellos
Dessert Choices to enjoy occasionally						
Fruit crumble	Grilled mango	Rice pudding	Grilled mango	Yam pie	Fertile Soul cookies	Chocolate strawberries
Beverage to sip on throughout the day						
Water	Licorice tea	Ginger tea	Chai tea	Kombucha	Lemonade	Ginseng tea

Dampness Meal Plan

Foods to resolve damp conditions: Aduki beans, alfalfa, anchovy, barley, cabbage, carrots, celery, corn, cranberries, garlic, green leafy vegetables, green tea, horseradish, jasmine tea, Job's tears, kidney bean, lemon, mackerel, marjoram, button mushrooms, mustard leaf, onion, parsley, pumpkin, plum, radish, rye, scallion, turnip.

Sunday	Monday	Tuesday	Wednesday	Thursday	Friday	Saturday
Breakfast						
Gourmet oatmeal	Poached egg on sprouted toast with avocado	Quinoa "Mother of Grains" and amaranth	Egg burrito	Miso soup	Conscious fritatta	Cocoberry pancakes
Snack						
Cranberry & walnuts	Hummus with rice crackers	Pear with nut butter	Sprouted loaf with nut butter	Miso soup	Dark leafy green wraps	Hummus with rice crackers
Lunch						
Curry vegetable soup add mighty greens	White bean stew	Lentil soup with coleslaw	Turkey meatballs with sauerkraut	Fertility soup	MIso soup with beet, pear & pistachio soup	Kidney beans, brown rice & mighty greens
Snack						
Roasted garlic brie with crackers	Savory quinoa bites with horseradish	Aduki bean stew	Shrimp cocktail with pumpkin pesto	Sushi rolls	Fajita nachos	Dolmas & babaganoush
Dinner						
Seafood dinner with brown rice	Salmon cakes and mighty greens	Pesto Spirals	Spaghetti squash Chicken marinara	Poached salmon Cruciferous crunch Moroccan pilaf	Tilapia	Pesto Spirals
Beverages to sip on throughout the day						
Water	Licorice tea	Ginger tea	Chai tea	Kombucha	Lemonade	Ginseng tea

KIDNEY IMBALANCES

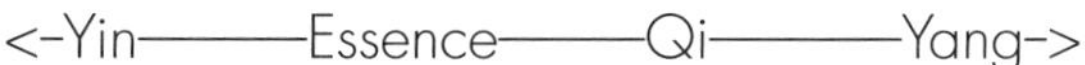

Lack of Cool - Lack of substance - Lack of energy - Lack of warmth

Kidney yin deficiency: low back or knee pain, prematurely grey hair, vaginal dryness, scanty cervical mucus, dark eye circles, hot flashes, fearful

Kidney yang deficiency: premenstrual low back pain, cold feet, low libido, frequent urination, and profuse vaginal discharge

Kidney essence deficiency: both yin and yang deficiencies

Western diagnoses: FSH, poor egg quality, recurrent miscarriage, luteal phase defect, advanced maternal age

Before we were born, our adrenal glands, kidneys, and reproductive organs developed together. The adrenal gland dominates this triad, squelching the proper functioning of the kidney and ovary when fear is present. Although fear represents self-preservation and survival instinct, the persistent state of fear indicates a kidney imbalance. It becomes pathologic when we feed it with daily stressors. Extremes of these emotions can also cause severe hormonal fluctuations in any endocrine organ, upsetting our reproductive capacity.

Lifestyle Recommendations

Reflective thought: journaling to inquire: what are we afraid of? How do we feel about ourselves? Where is fear holding you back in your life? What can you do in these areas to test your limits and expand your comfort zone? Who are we at our core?

Positive affirmations: I am whole perfect, complete, happy, healthy, harmonious strong, loving and powerful.

Meditation: Cultivating the habit of taking time out to listen to your inner voice. The sense organ related to the kidney energies is the ears. Consider listening to meditative music, while practicing deep-belly breathing.

Relaxation: Restorative yoga postures help to recalibrate the nervous system. Practicing savasana pose or "corpse pose" (the relaxation pose at the end of a yoga class) for five minutes each day does wonders for replenishing your entire system.

Salt soaks: A sea salt bath is marvelous for restoring kidney polarity and realigning our essence. Nightly foot soaks in Epson salt are also very restorative.

Abdominal self-massage: improves reproductive circulation, enhances kidney function and eliminates stress in the adrenals. With Kidney yang deficiency, apply heat to the abdomen between menstruation and ovulation.

Qi Gong: Use the microcosmic breath (circular breathing, down the front of the body and up the back of the body) visualizing the connection between the heart and uterus through the penetrating and conception meridians.

Swimming: The kidney and reproductive energies are related to the element of water. Swimming in salt water is particularly beneficial and restorative.

Walking: Because the focus is on replenishing kidney energies, it is preferable to avoid overexerting yourself and lean toward gently rejuvenating activities like walking.

Sleep: Aim to be asleep by 11pm each night and get 7-8 hours of rest to replenish your deepest reserves.

Kidney Essence Meal Plan

Foods to build reproductive essence: Adzuki bean, black bean, bee pollen, blue-green algae, chlorella, clams, corn, gelatin, kelp, legumes, lycium, millet, mulberry, organ meats, oysters, parsley, pumpkin seed, raspberry, royal jelly, spirulina, string bean, tofu, walnuts, wheat germ, wheat grass, wild rice, yam.

Sunday	Monday	Tuesday	Wednesday	Thursday	Friday	Saturday
Breakfast						
Mango Rice Pancakes	Sprouted Fertility Loaf	Gourmet Millet	Yam Congee	Quinoa "Mother of Grains"	Tofu Scramble	Cocoberry Pancakes
Snack						
Green Smoothie	Pumpkin seeds and goji berries	Banana Walnut Muffin	Green Smoothie	Sprouted Fertility Bread with jam	Berry Smoothie	Pumpkin seeds and goji berries
Lunch						
Black bean soup Brown rice	Fertility stew	Longevity Bone Soup	White Stew	Black beans Avocado Brown rice Greens	Coconut Red Rice with Mango & Cashews	Black beans Avocado Brown rice Greens
Snack						
Dolmas and Babaganoush	Black bean soup	Corn tortillas Guacamole	Shrimp cocktail with pumpkin seed pesto	White Bean Stew	Turkey meatballs with pineapple sauce	Hummus and toasted spelt pita
Dinner						
Broccoli Stir-Fry with Oyster Sauce and Brown Rice	Seafood Dinner with quinoa tabouli	Black bean burger, Kale Salad and Yam fries	Black bean and Yam Fajitas	Poached salmon Cruciferous crunch Moroccan pilaf	Salmon Cakes	Portobello Mushroom with Millet
Dessert choices to enjoy occasionally						
Berry Cobbler	Yam Pie	Rice pudding	Fruit Crumble	Rice Pudding	Fertile Soul cookies	Yam Pie Filling
Beverages to sip on throughout the day						
Water	Raspberry Tea	Nettles Tea	Kombucha	Sparkling Water	Mango Lassi	Pina Colado

Kidney Yang Meal Plan

Foods to generate warmth and vitality: Anchovy, aduki beans, anise, basil, beets, black beans, black pepper, caraway, cayenne, cherries, chestnut, chicken, chives, cinnamon bark, cloves, coriander, cumin, dates, dill, fennel, fenugreek seed, garlic, dried ginger, kidney, lamb, leeks, lentils, lobster, mussels, mustard leaf, mutton, nutmeg, oats, onions, peach, pine nuts, pistachio, quinoa, raspberry, rosemary, sage, scallions, shrimp, spelt, star anise, sweet brown rice, thyme, trout, turnip, walnuts.

Sunday	Monday	Tuesday	Wednesday	Thursday	Friday	Saturday
Breakfast						
"Omega 3" Benedict with Spinach	Quinoa "Mother of Grains"	Gourmet Oatmeal	Sprouted Fertility Loaf with Almond Butter	Quinoa "Mother of Grains"	Gourmet Oatmeal	Root Hash Trio
Snack						
Pistachio and Goji Berries	Sprouted Fertility Loaf with Nut Butter	Quinoa on the Go	Root Congee	Rice Crackers and Hummus	Goji Nut Muffins	Toasted Spelt Pita with Hummus
Lunch						
Black Beans, Avocado, Brown Rice and Spinach	Lentil Soup and Hawaii carrots	Black Bean Burger and Sauerkraut	Aduki Bean Stew and Brown Rice	Lentil Soup with Carrot and Broccoli Salad	Curried Root Stew with Pistachios	Aduki Bean Burger and Mighty Greens
Snack						
Roasted Garlic on Brie with Crackers	Corn Tortilla Chips and Guacamole	Dolmas and Babaganoush	Salmon Cakes	White Bean Stew	Turkey meatballs with pineapple sauce	Yam and Black Bean Salad
Dinner						
Roasted Chicken, Yam Casserole and Cruciferous Crunch	Yam and Black Bean Fajitas	Baked Salmon, Mighty Greens and Roasted Roots	Garlic Chicken, Brown Rice and Green Salad	Turkey Burgers, Yam Fries and Green Salad	Spaghetti Squash with Chicken Marinara	Brown Rice Pizza
Dessert choices to enjoy occasionally						
Chocolate Strawberries	Berry cobbler	Yam Pie	Goji Nut Muffins	Rice Pudding	Fertile Soul cookies	Fruit and Goat Yogurt
Beverage to sip on throughout the day						
Water	Chai Tea	Tulsi Tea	Raspberry Tea	Lemonade	Almost Soda	Chai Tea

Kidney Yin Meal Plan

Foods to cool and build reserves: Apple, asparagus, bananas, barley, bean sprouts, beets, blackberry, bulgur, cheese, chlorella, chickpeas, clam, crab, cuttlefish, duck, eggplant, eggs, honey, grapes, kidney bean, jellyfish, lemon, malt, mango, melon, milk, mulberry, organ meats, oyster, pea, pear, pineapples, pomegranate, pork, rabbit, raspberries, rice, seaweed, shellfish, spirulina, string bean, tofu, tomato, watermelon, yam.

Sunday	Monday	Tuesday	Wednesday	Thursday	Friday	Saturday
Breakfast						
Mango Rice Pancakes	Gourmet Oatmeal with Applesauce	Yam Congee	Miso Soup	Gourmet Oatmeal with Applesauce	Egg Buritto	Tofu Scramble
Snack						
Melon and Goat Yogurt	Berry Smoothie	Goji Nut Muffin	Green Smoothie	Sprouted Fertility Bread with Jam	Goji Nut Muffins	Granola and Goat Yogurt
Lunch						
Black Bean Soup with Brown Rice	Coconut Rice with Pepitas	Longevity Bone Soup	Black Bean Burgers with Red Bliss Potato Salad	Fertility Soup	Baked Salmon and Green Salad	Ratatouille with Shrimp and Brown Rice
Snack						
Dolmas and Babaganoush	Black Bean Soup	Corn Tortillas and Guacamole	Shrimp Cocktail with Pumpkin Pesto	Turkey meatballs with pineapple sauce	Corn Tortillas and Guacamole	Hummus and Toasted Spelt Pita
Dinner						
Seafood Dinner with Quinoa Tabouli	Poached Salmon with Brown Rice and Cruciferous Crunch	Black Bean Burger, Seaweed Salad, Yam Fries	Portobello Mushrooms with Millet	Broccoli Stir Fry with Oyster Sauce and Brown Rice	Black Bean and Yam Fajitas	Turkey Burgers and Asparagus Spears
Dessert choices to enjoy occasionally						
Grilled Mango	Blueberry Cobbler	Grilled mango	Yam Pie	Rice Crumble	Pineapple Slices	Pear with nut butter
Beverage to sip on throughout the day						
Water	Raspberry Tea	Mango Lassi	Nettle Tea	Peppermint Tea	Pina Colada	Goat Milk

LIVER QI STAGNATION AND EXCESS HEAT

Liver qi stagnation: depression, anger, premenstrual irritability, bloating, nipple discharge, painful menses

Excess heat: craves ice-cold drinks, dry throat and mouth, frequent thirst, short menstrual cycle, red acne

Western conditions: High FSH, hormonal imbalance, premenstrual syndrome, elevated prolactin, red skin rash/acne

Both Western and Eastern medicine agree that the liver's main functions include storage and filtration of blood, and metabolic activities including the metabolism of hormones. But Chinese medicine says that the Liver is also involved in the smooth flow and distribution of Blood. Liver Qi, the energy that fuels the liver's activities, is responsible for all transformations in the body, including ovulation, and for ensuring the smooth flow of emotions and Qi. When life unfolds in synergy with nature, our Liver energy flows freely. However, when we try to impose our will and refuse to accept what is, the energy becomes blocked and stagnant, resulting in liver obstruction: hormonal imbalances and overwhelming frustration and anger. Balancing the Liver can help to smooth our emotional energies and regenerate blood transmission to our source and spirit.

Lifestyle Recommendations

Release anger and resentment. Resolve feelings of frustration and judgment with forgiveness of self and others. Stagnant emotion can inhibit the qi mechanism. Use journaling or letter burning to release tension or scream out loud and punch a pillow.

Laugh out loud. Laughter is the cure for all ailments, so watch a funny movie or call a friend whose comedy brings you to tears, to release stuck internal feelings.

Breathe deep and relax. Circulating the breath immediately reduces stress levels by initiating the relaxation response and setting the stage for meditation.

Eye exercises: The sense organ of the liver is vision, thus we can use the eyes to clear out stuck memories; lying on your back, look up, look down, to the right, to the left, and make big circles in each direction. Repeated daily, this exercise can help reprogram thoughts, calm the nervous system and improve your vision.

Daily exercise will encourage the movement of qi (energy) and stimulate digestion and blood flow, flooding the body with feel-good endorphins. Choose an activity you enjoy and create a routine you can commit to that includes stretching, yoga and/or qi gong to help clear obstructions in the meridians and support your relaxation efforts.

Sleep: Aim to be asleep by 11pm each night and get 7-8 hours of rest to replenish your deepest reserves. In Chinese Medicine the hours between 11-1 am and 1-3 am are the corresponding times to the liver and gallbladder. Deep rest during these times promotes liver/gallbladder regeneration and supports hormonal balance.

Liver Qi Stagnation Meal Plan

Foods to move stagnant energy: Basil, caraway, cardamom, carrot, cayenne, chive, clove, coriander, dill seed, garlic, marjoram, mustard leaf, orange peel, peppermint, radish, rosemary, spearmint, star anise, tangerine peel, thyme, turmeric.

	Sunday	Monday	Tuesday	Wednesday	Thursday	Friday	Saturday
Breakfast	Pineapple French Toast (use egg replacer)	Tofu Scramble	Gourmet Oatmeal	Green Smoothie with Sprouted Fertility Toast and Ghee	Miso Soup	Yam Congee	Cocoberry pancakes
Snack	Goji Berries and Pumpkin Seeds	Green Smoothie	Rice Crackers and Hummus	Turkey, Avocado and Kale	Goji Berries and Pumpkin Seeds	Green Smoothie	Dark Leafy Green Wraps
Lunch	Carrot and Ginger Soup with Kale Salad	Lentil Soup with Carrot and Broccoli Salad	Butternut Squash Soup and Green Salad	Black Bean Burgers with Sauerkraut	White Bean Stew with Brown Rice and Coleslaw	Gazpacho with Beet, Pear and Pistachio Salad	Brown Rice Pasta with Pumpkin Seed Pesto
Appetizer	Corn Tortilla Chips with Guacamole	Dark Leafy Green Wraps	Savory Quinoa Bites with Horseradish	Dolmas and Babaganoush	Dark Leafy Green Wraps	White Bean Stew	Shrimp Cocktail with Pumpkin Seed Pesto
Dinner	Yam and Black Bean Fajitas	Garlic Chicken with Brown Rice and Hawaiian Carrots	Salmon Cakes, Mighty Greens and Roasted Roots	Turkey Burgers, Yam Fries and Green Salad	Poached Salmon with Pineapple Sauce	Brown Rice Pasta with Pumpkin Seeds Pesto	Curried Root Stew with Brown Rice
Dessert choices to enjoy occasionally	Grilled mango	Blueberry Cobbler	Grilled Mango	Pumpkin seeds and goji berries	Rice Pudding	Fertile Soul Cookies	Sweet potato pie
Beverage to sip on throughout the day	Water	Yogi Detox Tea	Milk Thistle Tea	Peppermint Tea	Kombucha	Wheat Grass	Chai Tea

BLOOD DEFICIENCY AND BLOOD STAGNATION

Blood deficiency: scant menses, dry skin, hair loss, poor nighttime vision, lightheaded

Blood stagnation: clotting in menses, dark spots in visual field, numbness in hands and feet, endometriosis, uterine fibroids, spider veins

Western conditions: amenorrhea, fibroids, endometriosis, and pelvic adhesions

The Chinese concept of the Heart encompasses the mind and spirit as well as the blood and circulatory system. The heart endows us with personality, and allows us peace. When other energies are imbalanced, the heart's functions become contracted. If too much of our energy is being consumed by desire, anxiety and fast living, our other organs contract and block the passage of the heart's transmission. This can manifest in loss of menstruation, insomnia, heart attack, or stroke. If there are emotional issues that affect the psyche, this may also influence the ability of the blood to nourish a developing fetus.

Lifestyle Recommendations

Gratitude and reverence practices: Visualize something that brings you a sense of gratitude and appreciation. Focus on that image. Feel your heart expanding and send the energies of appreciation and gratitude into your heart. Feel the sense of calm and unconditional love that is the heart's natural state of being. Keep a "gratitude journal" and make a list of five things that you are grateful for each day.

Meditate. Find a quiet corner in your home to create your space to sit and renew. Take the time to meditate, each day, closing your eyes and filling yourself with the positive vibrations of your sacred space.

Chant. There is a direct link between singing or chanting and the heart. Simply repeating the word OM sends healing vibrations to the heart, flooding you with feelings of joy.

Rest. Preserve boundaries and allow space to regain inner calm. Express your needs by nurturing yourself each day. Take a bath. Read a book. Meditate. Get an adequate amount of rest each night, going to sleep before 11 to support blood regeneration.

Qi gong and yoga: Use these practices to open your heart and gather "heavenly energies" through breath and movement. Place one hand on your heart and one hand on your belly to connect your life-giving energies.

Dance. Life is created through our bodies. We express ourselves through art, dance, and creativity. Color, paint, dance and flow to your own rhythm.

Sleep: Aim to be asleep by 11pm each night and get 7-8 hours of rest to experience deep calm and centeredness in your daily life.

Blood Stagnation Meal Plan

Foods to move stagnant blood: Abalone, beets, bilberry, Brussels sprout, chestnut, chili pepper, chive, crab, cucumbers, dark green vegetables, eggplant, evening primrose oil, fish and fish oil, hawthorn berry, kelp, lemon, lime, linseed oil, mustard leaf, nuts and seed oils, onion, peach, saffron, scallion, seaweed, spirulina, squid, sturgeon, turnips, vinegar.

Sunday	Monday	Tuesday	Wednesday	Thursday	Friday	Saturday
Breakfast						
Quinoa "Mother of Grains" with peaches	Egg Burrito	Gourmet Oatmeal with Flaxseed	Green Smoothie with Fertility Sprouted Loaf and Ghee	Miso Soup	Root Congee	Coco-berry pancakes
Snack						
Goji Berries and Pumpkin Seeds	Green Smoothie	Rice Crackers and Hummus	Turkey, Avocado and Kale Wraps	Goji Berries and Pumpkin Seeds	Green Smoothie	Dark Leafy Green Wraps
Lunch						
Carrot Ginger Soup with Seaweed Salad	Coconut Dahl with Brown Rice	Butternut Squash Soup with Mighty Greens	Black Bean Burgers with Broccoli	White Bean Stew with Brown Rice and Coleslaw	Gazpacho with Beet, Pear and Pistachio Salad	Curry Stew with Spinach Salad
Snack						
Corn Tortillas with guacamole	Dark Leafy Green Wraps	Salmon Cakes	Dolmas and Babaganoush	Dark Leafy Green Wraps	White Bean Stew	Shrimp Cocktail and Pumpkin Seed Pesto
Dinner						
Yam and Aduki Bean Fajitas	Broccoli Stir Fry with Oyster Sauce with Brown Rice	Salmon Cakes, Mighty Greens and Roasted Roots	Eggplant Parmesan, Grateful Greens	Poached Salmon with Pineapple Sauce	Brown Rice Pasta with Pumpkin Seed Pesto	Seafood Dinner
Dessert choices to enjoy occasionally						
Fertile Soul cookies	Peach Cobbler	Grilled Mango	Crispy Treats	Rice pudding	Fertile Soul cookies	Goji nut muffins
Beverage to sip on throughout the day						
Water	Yogi Detox Tea	Milk Thistle Tea	Ginger Tea	Hot Water with Lemon	Chamomile Tea	Chai Tea

Blood Deficiency Meal Plan

Foods to build and Nourish Blood: Aduki bean, apricot, beef, beetroot, blackberries, bone marrow, eggs, cuttlefish, dark leafy greens, date, dandelion, fig, grape, kidney bean, liver, hormone-free meat and liver, microalgae, nettle, octopus, oyster, parsley, raspberry, sardine, spinach, spirulina, sweet rice, watercress.

	Sunday	Monday	Tuesday	Wednesday	Thursday	Friday	Saturday
Breakfast	Tofu Scramble	Gourmet Oatmeal with Apple Sauce	Conscious Frittata	Quinoa "Mother of Grains"	Egg Burrito	Root Congee	Tofu Scramble
Snack	Banana Walnut Bread	Sesame Mochi Balls	Berry Smoothie	Granola and Goat Yogurt	Trail Mix	Dark Leafy Greens	Green Smoothie
Lunch	Coconut Rice with Mango and Cashews	White Bean Stew with Brown Rice	Turkey Burgers with Beet, pistachio and pear salad	Fertility Stew	Black Bean Burgers with Mighty Greens	Longevity Soup	Black beans Avocado Brown rice Greens
Snack	Dolmas and Babaganoush	Dark Leafy Green Wraps	Fajita Nachos	Corn Tortillas and guacamole	Fertility Stew	Turkey meatballs with pineapple sauce	Black bean Burger Bites
Dinner	Tri-Tip, Yam Casserole and Mighty Greens	Broccoli Stir Fry with Oyster Sauce with Brown Rice	Meat Chili with Brown Rice	Poached Salmon, Cruciferous Crunch and Quinoa	Tri-Tip, Yam Casserole and Mighty Greens	Stuffed Portobello Mushroom	Spaghetti Squash with Chicken Marinara
Dessert choices to enjoy occasionally	Grilled Mango	Blueberry Cobbler	Grilled mango	Yam Pie	Rice Pudding	Fertile Soul cookies	Goji nut muffins
Beverage to sip on throughout the day	Water	Peppermint Tea	Honeysuckle Tea	Milk Thistle Tea	Lemonade	Goat Milk	Sparkling Grapefruit

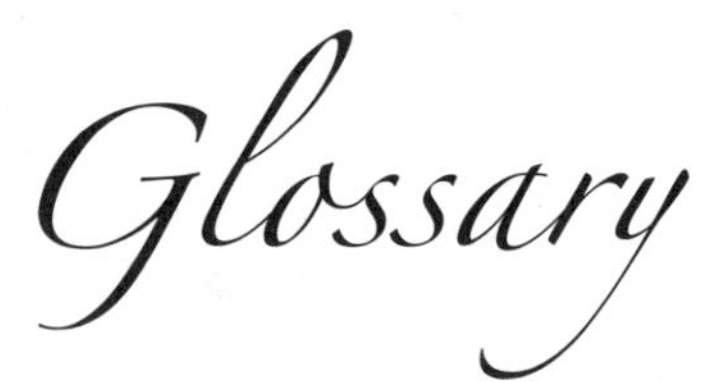

A	Fertility Benefit	Recipe Glossary
Almonds	• Protein source • Contains zinc and Vitamin E, which support the health of the uterine lining and placenta in pregnancy • Ayurvedic choice for building "ojas" – spiritual and reproductive ability	**Breakfast** Quinoa Mother of Grains Granola Goji Nut Muffins Pineapple French Toast **Beverages** Nut Milk Berry Smoothie Chai Tea Tea Chino Almond Milk Hotta Chocolatta **Appetize and Snack** Fruits and nuts Shrimp skewers with pumpkin pesto Dark leafy green wraps **Salad** Grateful greens **Main Attraction** Eggplant casserole Pad thai Seafood dinner **Desserts** Randine's popcorn Crispy treats Rice pudding Berry cobbler Sweet potato pie
Apples	• Cooling in nature; nourishes yin • Benefits low blood sugar conditions and emotional depression	**Breakfast** Applesauce Oatmeal Sprouted Fertility Loaf with Nut butters **Beverages** Green smoothie **Appetize and Snack** Fruits and Nuts **Soup** Butternut Squash Bisque **Salad** Waldorf with light goat dressing Seaweed salad

Asparagus	• Encourages yin receptivity and compassion, the very nature of fertility • Softens difficult menses	**Sides** Ginger Sesame Asparagus
Avocado	• Supports the liver • Excellent source of monounsaturated fat and protein • Rich in copper to promote red blood cell production; lecithin to enhance brain function • Vitamin E source for healthy sperm and cervical mucous	**Breakfast** Avocado and egg on toast Egg burrito Omega 3 benedict over spinach **Appetize and Snack** Green smoothie Guacamole Sushi **Salad** Grateful greens Spinach salad **Main Attraction** Yam and black bean fajitas Pumpkin Pesto Pasta
B Basil	• Vitalizes energy flow • Resolves PMS, blood clotting, fibroids, and release stuck emotions	**Breakfast** Fritatta **Appetize and Snack** Shrimp cocktail with pumpkin pesto **Salad** Spinach salad with omega pesto dressing Red Bliss salad Pasta Bruschetta **Sides** Ratatouille **Main Attraction** Brown rice pizza with pesto sauce Pesto spirals Spaghetti squash marinara
Beets	• The color red indicates its benefits to both the heart and the blood • Stimulates more frequent menstruation in lengthy cycles or amenorrhea	**Breakfast** Root hash trio **Salad** Roasted beet, pistachio and pear salad **Sides** Roasted rosemary roots

Bell peppers	• Rich in vitamin C • Promotes circulation of qi and blood throughout the body	**Breakfast** Tofu Scramble **Appetize and Snack** Fajita Nachos with Salsa and Guacamole **Sides** Ratatouille Loaded Yams with Mighty greens **Main Attraction** Yam and black bean fajitas Garlic Cashew Chicken
Black beans	• Fortifies the kidneys and reproductive function	**Soup** Black bean soup Fertility Stew **Salad** Southwestern black bean salad **Sides** Simple Beans **Main Attraction** Black bean burgers Yam and black bean fajitas
Black sesame seeds	• Builds blood and yin; supporting reproductive function	**Breakfast** Root Congee **Appetize and Snack** Fruits and nuts Sushi **Salad** Coleslaw with Deb's simple salad dressing Seaweed salad **Sides** Ginger Sesame Asparagus **Main Attraction** Black bean burgers
Blueberries	• Nourishes kidney Yin • Supports the resolution of "urinary, sexual and reproductive imbalances"	**Breakfast** Gourmet Oatmeal Coco-berry pancakes **Beverages** Berry Smoothie **Appetize and Snack** Fruits and nuts **Desserts** Berry cobbler

Broccoli	• Supports metabolism of excess estrogens with DIM • Rich in cancer-preventing phytochemicals • Contains high levels of vitamin A, vitamin C, sulfur, iron, and B vitamins • Promotes bright eyes	**Appetize and Snack** Fajita Nachos with Salsa and Guacamole Turkey meatballs with pineapple sauce **Soups** Fertility Stew **Sides** Broccoli with oyster sauce Cruciferous crunch **Main Attraction** Turkey Meatloaf
Brown rice	• Contains more than 70 antioxidants • Promotes cell regeneration and blood circulation • Strengthens the immune system • Calms an anxious or depressed mind	**Breakfast** Cooking Whole Grains Yam Scones **Appetize and Snack** Dolmas with Babaganoush Sushi **Salad** Pasta Bruschetta **Sides** Moroccan pilaf Coconut rice with pepitas Pineapple Ginger Fried rice **Main Attraction** Pad thai Brown rice pizza Pesto Spirals **Desserts** Crispy treats Fertile Soul Cookies Sweet potato pie Coconut Rice pudding
C Cabbage	• Detoxifies the liver • Alleviates symptoms of pre-menstrual tension, irritability, headaches, and breast tenderness at ovulation	**Appetize and Snack** Dark Leafy green wraps **Soup** **Salad** Cole slaw with Deb's simple salad dressing **Sides** Sauerkraut

Carrots	• Abundant in beta-carotene • Helps alkalize the blood	**Appetize and Snack** Dark Leafy green wraps Sushi **Soup** Fertility stew **Sides** Hawaiian Carrots **Main Attraction** Veggie burgers
Cardamom, cinnamon, cloves	• Stimulates sexual energy • Invigorates blood flow; moves stagnant energy, alleviating conditions of fibroids, endometriosis and PMS. • Helps regulate insulin resistance, important in PCOS	**Breakfast** Applesauce Quinoa mother of grains Root congee Granola Sprouted Fertility Loaf with Nut butters Yam Scones Pineapple French Toast **Beverages** Chai Tea Hotta Chocolatta **Sides** Moroccan pilaf Baked Butternut Squash **Main Attraction** Tri-tip **Desserts** Banana walnut bread Crispy treats Sweet potato pie Coconut Rice pudding Chocolate mousse
Chamomile	• Calming • Gently detoxifies the liver • Relieves headaches, anxiety, and menstrual cramps	**Beverages** Tea infusions with fresh herbs
Chlorophyll (greens and algae sources)	• Purifies and reduces inflammation • Called "the blood of plant life" • Supplement in cases of PCOS to stabilize blood sugar levels	**Breakfast** Root Hash Trio **Appetize and Snack** Fajita Nachos with Salsa and Guacamole Turkey meatballs with pineapple sauce Dark Leafy green wraps **Salad** Seaweed salad Grateful Greens with raspberry vinaigrette

Chlorophyll (cont'd)		Caesar Spinach with creamy pesto dressing Waldorf with a light goat dressing **Sides** Cruciferous crunch Cauli-mash Ginger Sesame Asparagus Loaded Yams with Mighty greens **Main Attraction** Turkey Meatloaf Garlic cashew chicken Yam and black bean fajitas Pesto Spirals
Chocolate	• Healthy monounsaturated fat source • Smell promotes the relaxation response • Flavanoids known to help elevate mood, promote blood flow, ease inflammation and inhibit the formation of blood clots • Contains arginine that increases blood flow to the uterus and ovaries	**Beverages** Hotta Chocolatta **Desserts** Crispy treats Fertile Soul Cookies Berry cobbler Chocolate mousse
Coconut	• Supports digestive function • Strengthens the reproductive organs and the liver's ability to process hormones • Increases semen as well as Yin fluids, including cervical mucus	**Breakfast** Coco-berry pancakes Beverages Coconut Milk Pina Colada **Appetize and Snack** Fruits and nuts **Sides** Moroccan pilaf Coconut rice with pepitas Coconut Dahl **Desserts** Crispy treats Fertile Soul Cookies Coconut Rice pudding
Corn	• A heart-nourishing grain that promotes vitality in the sexual organs	**Breakfast** Cooking Whole Grains Root Hash Trio **Salad** Southwestern black bean salad **Sides** Broccoli with oyster sauce **Main Attraction** Yam and black bean fajitas **Desserts** Randine's popcorn

Cruciferous vegetables (kale, cauliflower, broccoli, Brussels sprouts, bok choy, cabbage)	• Contain di-indolymethane (DIM), a compound that stimulates more efficient use of estrogen by increasing the metabolism of estradiol • Combats breast pain, weight gain, breast and uterine cancer, moodiness and low libido	**Appetize and Snack** Fajita Nachos with Salsa and Guacamole Turkey meatballs with pineapple sauce **Soup** Fertility Stew **Salad** Cole slaw with Deb's simple salad dressing **Sides** Cruciferous crunch Cauli-mash Simple Beans Sauerkraut **Main Attraction** Turkey Meatloaf
E Eggplant	• A rich source of bioflavanoids • An ideal treatment for stagnant blood in the uterus • Resolves repressed emotion in both the uterus and liver • Note: do not use in pregnancy due to its hemostatic qualities	**Appetize and Snack** Dolmas with Babaganoush **Sides** Ratatouille **Main Attraction** Eggplant Parmesan
Eggs	• Nourishes and builds the blood • Source of protein and vitamin B12	**Breakfast** Yam Scones Goji Berry Nut Muffins Egg Burrito The Conscious Fritatta "Omega 3 Benedict" over Spinach with Hollandaise Sauce Coco-berry pancakes **Main Attraction** Turkey Meatloaf Seafood dinner Eggplant Parmesan **Desserts** Banana walnut bread
F Flaxseed	• Benefits digestion and all reproductive function • Provides omega-3s helpful for blood flow, morphology, mobility	**Breakfast** Gourmet oatmeal Quinoa mother of grains Granola **Beverages** Berry Smoothie **Appetize and Snack** Fruits and nuts **Salad** Coleslaw with Deb's simple salad dressing **Desserts** Berry cobbler

Fruit	• Alkalizes and cleanses the body • Contain many beneficial nutrients, minerals, enzymes and fiber	**Breakfast** Applesauce Sprouted Fertility Loaf with Nut butters Gourmet Oatmeal Coco-berry pancakes Pineapple French Toast Quinoa mother of grains **Beverages** Green smoothie Berry Smoothie Mango Lhassi Pina Colada **Appetize and Snack** Fruits and nuts Turkey meatballs with pineapple sauce **Salad** Beet, Pistachio, Pear Salad Cucumber, Kale and Seaweed Salad Waldorf with a light goat dressing Red Bliss salad **Sides** Coconut rice with pepitas Pineapple Ginger Fried rice Hawaiian Carrots **Main Attraction** Poached Salmon with Pineapple Sauce **Desserts** Banana walnut bread Chocolate covered strawberries Berry cobbler Grilled mango
G Garbanzo beans	• Contains more iron than any other legume, an important ingredient for building blood in scant or missing periods and conditions of anemia. • Good source of healthy fats	**Appetize and Snack** Hummus
Garlic	• Vitalizes energy flow to alleviate PMS, blood clotting, fibroids, and release stuck emotions • Selenium helps with male fertility and miscarriage prevention • Strengthens immune system • B6 promotes hormonal balance	**Breakfast** Tofu Scramble **Appetize and Snack** Dolmas with Babaganoush Fajita Nachos with Salsa and Guacamole Roasted Garlic on Goat Brie Turkey meatballs with pineapple sauce **Soup** White bean stew Black bean soup Cream of vegetable soup Fertility Stew

Garlic (cont'd)		Gazpacho Lentil **Salad** Southwestern black bean salad Caesar Spinach with creamy pesto dressing **Sides** Coconut Dahl Roasted rosemary roots Loaded Yams with Mighty greens Ratatouille Cauli-mash Loaded Yams with Mighty greens **Main Attraction** Tri-tip Black bean burgers Turkey Meatloaf Garlic cashew chicken Stuffed Portobello Yam and black bean fajitas Pesto Spirals Spaghetti squash with marinara
Ginger	• Supports digestion • Stimulates menses • Useful in long cycles and amenorrhea	**Breakfast** Yam Scones **Beverages** Tea infusions with fresh herbs Chai Tea **Appetize and Snack** Dolmas with Babaganoush Sushi **Soup** Butternut Squash Bisque Carrot Ginger **Sides** Broccoli with oyster sauce Pineapple Ginger Fried rice **Main Attraction** Garlic cashew chicken
Goat milk products	• Important source of calcium to support the nervous system, bones, and blood • Contains tryptophan to promote relaxation • An easily digestible source of full fat dairy to meet the latest recommendations from the Nurses Study findings	**Breakfast** Quinoa mother of grains Egg Burrito **Beverages** Berry Smoothie Chai Tea Tea Chino Hotta Chocolatta Mango Lhassi **Appetize and Snack** Fajita Nachos with Salsa and Guacamole

Goat milk products (cont'd)		Roasted Garlic on Goat Brie **Soup** Cream of vegetable **Salad** Greek with goat feta vinaigrette Spinach with creamy pesto dressing Pasta Bruschetta Waldorf with a light goat dressing **Sides** Cauli-mash Baked Butternut Squash **Main Attraction** Stuffed Portobello Mushrooms Eggplant Parmesan **Desserts** Grilled mango Sweet potato pie Coconut Rice pudding
Goji berries	• Nourishes the blood • Helps to balance blood sugar levels • Fortifies sexual energy, considered an aphrodisiac in Chinese Medicine	**Breakfast** Root congee Goji Nut Muffins **Appetize and Snack** Dolmas with Babaganoush **Sides** Moroccan pilaf **Main Attraction** Roasted chicken with stuffing **Desserts** Fertile Soul Cookies Coconut Rice pudding
Grains	• Helps to overcome sugar cravings supports digestion, mood, energy levels and restful sleep • Fosters a peaceful mind and induce a state of receptivity • Contains Vitamin A and E that help with hormonal balance, healthy egg and sperm quality	**Breakfast** Cooking Whole Grains Gourmet Oatmeal Root congee **Appetize and Snack** Dolmas with Babaganoush Sushi Savory Quinoa Bites with Hummus **Salad** Pasta Bruschetta Quinoa tabouli **Sides** Moroccan pilaf Coconut rice with pepitas Pineapple Ginger Fried rice **Main Attraction** Pad thai Brown rice pizza Pesto Spirals

Grains (cont'd)		**Desserts** Berry cobbler Crispy treats Fertile Soul Cookies Sweet potato pie Coconut Rice pudding
Greens	• Contains abundant iron and chlorophyll, an essential element in a fertility-enhancing diet • Note: for the most benefits choose the darkest greens available	**Breakfast** Root Hash Trio Beverages Green Smoothie **Appetize and Snack** Dark Leafy green wraps with Raita **Soup** White bean stew Fertility Stew Green puree **Salad** Seaweed salad Grateful Greens with raspberry vinaigrette Caesar Spinach with creamy pesto dressing Waldorf with a light goat dressing **Sides** Loaded Yams with Mighty greens **Main Attraction** Yam and black bean fajitas Pesto Spirals
K Kombucha	• Contains many beneficial probiotics, enzymes, vitamins, and amino acids • Helps restore healthy flora balance to the gut and contributes to improved digestion, immunity, metabolism, cellular development and liver function • Believed to balance hormones and improve fertility in men and women	**Beverages** Kombucha
L Lemon/Lime	• Vitamin C improves sperm quality and supports ovulation	**Beverages** Lemonade Limeade Almost Soda **Appetize and Snack** Green Smoothie Dolmas with Babaganoush Fajita Nachos with Salsa and Guacamole **Salad** Beet, pistachio, pear salad with balsamic

Lemon/Lime (cont'd)		Southwestern black bean salad Caesar Greek with goat feta vinaigrette **Main Attraction** Pad Thai Pesto Spirals
M Mango	• Builds yin fluids • Replenishes adrenal and reproductive system	**Beverages** Tea infusions with fresh herbs Mango Lhassi **Sides** Coconut rice with pepitas Desserts Grilled mango
Milk thistle	• Helps to detoxify the liver • Helps with PMS symptoms	**Beverages** Tea infusions with fresh herbs
Mushrooms	• Strengthens the entire body • Builds immunity	**Breakfast** Root Hash Trio Tofu Scramble **Beverages** Kombucha **Soup** Miso Fertility Stew **Salad** Grateful Greens with raspberry vinaigrette **Main Attraction** Stuffed Portobello Mushrooms
N Nettles	• Helps increase energy and nourishing the blood	**Breakfast** Mochi with nettles Sprouted Fertility Loaf with Nut butters **Beverages** Tea infusions with fresh herbs
Nuts	• Contains essential fatty acids and vitamin E, a nerve protector and immune-enhancing antioxidant	**Breakfast** Goji Berry Nut Muffins Root congee Gourmet Oatmeal Granola Yam Scones Pineapple French Toast **Appetize and Snack** Fruits and nuts **Salad** Grateful Greens with raspberry vinaigrette Spinach with creamy pesto dressing Waldorf with a light goat dressing **Sides** Moroccan pilaf

Nuts (cont'd)		Broccoli with oyster sauce Baked Butternut Squash Sweet yam and walnut casserole **Main Attraction** Stuffed Portobello Mushrooms **Desserts** Banana walnut bread Coconut Rice pudding
O Oats (rolled)	• Stabilizes blood sugar and energy levels • Contains Vitamin A and E that help with hormonal balance, healthy egg and sperm	**Breakfast** Cooking Whole Grains Gourmet Oatmeal **Desserts** Berry cobbler
Olive oil	• Healthy cooking oil • Omega 3 benefits blood flow, morphology, mobility and all reproductive function	**Breakfast** Yam Scones Egg Burrito Conscious Fritatta Root Hash Trio Tofu Scramble Pineapple French Toast Coco-berry pancakes Appetize and Snack Dolmas with Babaganoush Shrimp Cocktail with Pumpkin pesto Fajita Nachos with Salsa and Guacamole Turkey meatballs with pineapple sauce **Soup** White bean stew Black bean stew Butternut squash bisque Fertility Stew Gazpacho Green puree Lentil Carrot Ginger **Salad** Grateful Greens with raspberry vinaigrette Caesar Greek with goat feta vinaigrette Spinach with creamy pesto dressing Waldorf with a light goat dressing **Sides** Moroccan pilaf Yam fries Coconut Dal Quinoa tabouli Roasted rosemary roots

Olive oil (cont'd)		**Main Attraction** Tri-tip Veggie burgers Turkey Meatloaf Roasted chicken with stuffing Poached Salmon with Pineapple Sauce Brown rice pizza Tilapia with sautéed spinach Yam and black bean fajitas Pesto Spirals Spaghetti squash with marinara
Oysters	• Aphrodisiac • Helps build blood and yin • Zinc helps with sperm and egg production	**Main Attraction** Seafood dinner
P Parsley	• Contains vitamin A, chlorophyll, calcium, sodium and magnesium • Fortifies the adrenals, a paired organ of the reproductive system	**Appetize and Snack** Dolmas with Babaganoush **Soup** Butternut Squash Bisque **Salad** Red Bliss salad **Sides** Yam fries **Main Attraction** Ratatouille Spaghetti squash with marinara
Peppermint	• Relieves symptoms of PMS and other stagnations in the body	**Beverages** Tea infusions with fresh herbs
Pineapple	• Contains bromelain, an enzyme helpful in promoting implantation	**Breakfast** Pineapple French Toast **Beverages** Pina Colada **Appetize and Snack** Fruits and nuts Turkey meatballs with pineapple sauce **Salad** Red Bliss salad **Sides** Pineapple Ginger Fried rice Hawaiian Carrots **Main Attraction** Poached Salmon with Pineapple Sauce

Pumpkin seeds	• Omega 3 fatty acids for blood flow, morphology, mobility and all reproductive function and zinc, essential for proper hormone processing and sperm production	**Breakfast** Granola Sprouted Fertility Loaf with Nut butters Goji Berry Nut Muffins **Appetize and Snack** Fruits and nuts Shrimp Cocktail with Pumpkin pesto **Salad** Spinach with creamy pesto dressing **Sides** Coconut rice with pepitas **Main Attraction** Seafood dinner Yam and black bean fajitas Pesto Spirals **Desserts** Fertile Soul Cookies Coconut Rice pudding
Pungent spices	• Cleanse the liver • Help to regulate the menstrual cycle	**Breakfast** Tofu Scramble **Appetize and Snack** Hummus **Soup** Black bean soup Cream of vegetable Fertility Stew Gazpacho Chili Curried Root Stew Lentil **Salad** Greek with goat feta vinaigrette
Q Quinoa	• Packs 16% more protein than any other grain • Contains manganese, magnesium and iron in addition to all 9 essential amino acids.	**Breakfast** Cooking Whole Grains Quinoa "Mother of Grains" Sprouted Fertility Loaf with Nut butters **Appetize and Snack** Savory Quinoa Bites with Hummus **Salad** Quinoa tabouli
R Red clover	• Contains Vitamin B, thiamine, Vitamin C and Calcium • Helps to relax the nervous system and alkalize cervical mucous, creating an ideal PH balance in the uterus • Helps to regulate the menstrual cycle	**Breakfast** Sprouted Fertility Loaf with Nut butters **Beverages** Tea infusions with fresh herbs

Red meat	• Source of iron to build blood and energy • Important in cases of anemia or amenorrhea • Can help support ovulation • Note: always choose lean grass-fed, hormone-free varieties	**Main Attraction** Tri-tip
Red raspberry	• Raspberries enrich and cleanse the blood of toxins and regulate the menstrual cycle. • Tones the uterus, support conception and prevent pregnancy complications	**Breakfast** Quinoa mother of grains Coco-berry pancakes **Salad** Grateful Greens with raspberry vinaigrette **Desserts** Berry cobbler Grilled mango Red raspberry tea **Beverages** Tea infusions with fresh herbs
Root vegetables	• "Grow in cold climates and contain minerals and other elements that make it possible to survive in harsh weather and under snow." • With a multitude of vitamins, the essence of reproductive capability is fortified	**Breakfast** Root Hash Trio **Soup** Longevity Soup Butternut Squash Bisque Cream of Vegetable Soup Fertility Stew Curried Root Stew Lentil Carrot Ginger **Salad** Red Bliss salad **Sides** Roasted rosemary roots **Main Attraction** Yam and black bean fajitas Spaghetti squash with marinara
Royal Jelly	• Strengthens reproductive function • Improves egg quality • Rich in amino acids, vitamins, and enzymes, royal jelly helps the queen lay millions of eggs and live longer than the worker bee.	**Beverages** Mango Lassi
S Salmon	• Omega 3 source helpful for blood flow, morphology, mobility and all reproductive function	**Breakfast** "Omega 3 Benedict" over Spinach with Hollandaise Sauce **Main Attraction** Poached Salmon with Pineapple Sauce Salmon Cakes

Sardines	• A source of protein that builds the yin reserves and supports blood circulation • Omega 3 source helpful for blood flow, morphology, mobility and all reproductive function	**Salad** Caesar
Seaweeds	• Healthy minerals, vitamins, amino acids, calcium, iodine, iron, high in fiber and A, B, C, D, E, and K vitamin complexes. • A source of chlorophyll; seaweed revitalizes our essence; fertility and sexual energy	**Salad** Seaweed salad **Soup** Miso **Sides** Simple Beans Sauerkraut
Shrimp	• Enhances yang, supporting progesterone levels essential for maintaining pregnancy and also reducing spotting between periods	**Appetize and Snack** Shrimp Cocktail with Pumpkin pesto
Spinach	• Rich in iron and chlorophyll • Folic acid source to support healthy neural development in pregnancy • Build and purify the blood • Particularly beneficial in cases of scanty blood flow, short cycles and amenorrhea	**Breakfast** "Omega 3 Benedict" over Spinach with Hollandaise Sauce **Salad** Spinach with creamy pesto dressing **Main Attraction** Stuffed Portobello Mushrooms Tilapia with sautéed spinach
T Tea	• Preferentially dilates blood vessels in the body supporting flow	**Beverages** Tea infusions with fresh herbs Chai tea
Tofu	• Yin building; cooling • Vegetarian protein source • Good source of B vitamins and minerals, including calcium, phosphorous, iron, sodium, and potassium	**Breakfast** Tofu Scramble **Soup** Fertility Stew Miso **Desserts** Chocolate mousse
Tomatoes	• Cooling and nourishing to the adrenals, reproductive organs and kidneys • Produce an alkalizing reaction in the body and help purify the blood.	**Appetize and Snack** Fajita Nachos with Salsa and Guacamole **Soup** White Bean Stew Cream of Vegetable Soup Fertility Stew Gazpacho **Salad** Southwestern black bean salad

Tomatoes (cont'd)		Grateful Greens with raspberry vinaigrette Greek with goat feta vinaigrette Pasta Bruschetta Quinoa tabouli **Sides** Ratatouille **Main Attraction** Turkey Meatloaf Stuffed Portobello Eggplant Parmesan Spaghetti squash with marinara
Turkey	• Tryptophan and B vitamins reduce the impact of stress, thereby supporting fertility	**Appetize and Snack** Turkey meatballs with pineapple sauce **Salad** Spinach with creamy pesto dressing **Sides** Loaded Yams with Mighty greens **Main Attraction** Turkey Meatloaf
Turmeric	• Reduces inflammation • Helps to detoxify the liver • Sends blood flow to the uterus and ovaries	**Breakfast** Tofu Scramble **Appetize and Snack** Shrimp Cocktail with Pumpkin pesto Savory Quinoa Bites with Hummus **Sides** Moroccan pilaf Cauli-mash **Main Attraction** Tilapia with sautéed spinach
W Walnuts	• Contain omegas, which help move stagnations of the blood as in conditions of clotted menses and fibroids.	**Breakfast** Gourmet Oatmeal Granola Yam Scones **Appetize and Snack** Fruits and nuts **Salad** Grateful Greens with raspberry vinaigrette Spinach with creamy pesto dressing Waldorf with a light goat dressing **Sides** Broccoli with oyster sauce Baked Butternut Squash Sweet yam and walnut casserole **Main Attraction** Stuffed Portobello Mushrooms **Desserts** Banana walnut bread Coconut Rice pudding

Wheat grass	• A high protein cereal grass high • Contains B vitamins and anti-inflammatory properties that also promote cell regeneration. • Helps detoxify the liver, reduce FSH, regulate menstrual cycles	**Appetize and Snack** Green Smoothie
Y Yams	• Yin and Qi building • High in Vitamin A • One study conducted in a small village in Nigeria showed that high yam consumption may be the reason that women, in this tribe, produce multiple fertile eggs and ultimately twins. • Yams are quite sweet and should be avoided in conditions of PCOS. • Note: Most yams found in North America are actually sweet potatoes. Find the white variety at African specialty food stores	**Breakfast** Yam Scones Root Congee **Soup** Fertility Stew Curried Root Stew **Salad** Southwestern Black Bean Salad **Sides** Yam fries Roasted rosemary roots Sweet yam and walnut casserole Loaded Yams with Mighty greens **Main Attraction** Yam and black bean fajitas **Desserts** Sweet potato pie (made with yams)

Notes

CHINESE MEDICINE AND THE REPRODUCTIVE SYSTEM

1. Pitchford, Paul. Healing with Whole Foods: Asian Traditions and Modern Nutrition. Berkeley, CA: North Atlantic Books, 2002; 363.

2. Ibid., 580

BASIC GUIDELINES

3. Willett, Walter C., Patrick J. Skerrett, and Jorge E. Chavarro. The Fertility Diet. New York: McGraw-Hill Companies, The, 2007; 109

4. Price, Madelon. "Aspartame causes infertility." David Oliver Rietz's Dorway to Discovery. 21 Mar. 1997. 28 Oct. 2008 http://www.dorway.com/betty/drprice.html

5. Dellorto, Danielle. "Study: Caffeine may boost miscarriage risk." CNN.com/health. 21 Jan. 2008. 28 Oct. 2008. http://www.cnn.com/2008/health/conditions/01/21hfh.caffeine.miscarriage/index.html

6. Pitchford, Paul. Healing with Whole Foods: Asian Traditions and Modern Nutrition. Berkeley, CA: North Atlantic Books, 2002; 27

7. Pitchford, Paul. "Healing with Whole Foods." PowerPoint presentation. Heartwood Institute, Garberville, CA. August 2006

8. Pitchford, Paul. Healing with Whole Foods: Asian Traditions and Modern Nutrition. Berkeley, CA: North Atlantic Books, 2002; 26-30 and 45

9. Willett, Walter C., Patrick J. Skerrett, and Jorge E. Chavarro. The Fertility Diet. New York: McGraw-Hill Companies, The, 2007; 73

10. Pitchford, Paul. Healing with Whole Foods: Asian Traditions and Modern Nutrition. Berkeley, CA: North Atlantic Books, 2002; 164

11. Ibid., 178

11a. Tiberi, Dr. Robin Saraswati. "Nourishing Life." 19 Mar 2010. http://nourishinglife.com/

ALIGNING WITH THE CYCLES OF THE MOON

12. Lewis, Randine A. The Infertility Cure : The Ancient Chinese Wellness Program for Getting Pregnant and Having Healthy Babies. Boston: Little Brown & Company, 2005; 22

13. Ibid., 23

BREAK THE FAST

14. Pitchford, Paul. "Subject: from Paul Pitchford." Email to Kathryn Flynn. 1 Mar. 2009.

15. "Egg, whole, raw, fresh." Agricultural Research Service (ARS) Mar. 28 2009 http://www.ars.usda.gov/main/site_main.htm?modecode=12354500

16. University of Surrey. "Two-egg diet cracks cholesterol issue." Physorg.com. 28 Apr. 2008. http://www.physorg.com/news139156140.html August 28th, 2008

17. Pitchford, Paul. Healing with Whole Foods: Asian Traditions and Modern Nutrition. Berkeley, CA: North Atlantic Books, 2002; 459

18. Ibid., 617

19. Ibid., 470

20. Ibid., 477

21. Pitchford, Paul. "Healing with Whole Foods." Heartwood Institute, Garberville, CA. August 2006.

22. Weed, Susan S. Wise Woman Herbal for the Childbearing Year. Woodstock, NY: Ashtree, 1986; 2.

23. A., Misi. "Eat More Yam And Give Birth To Twins!" African Loft. 12 Nov. 2007. 28 Oct. 2008 http://www.africanloft.com/eat-more-yam-and-give-birth-to-twins/

24. Pitchford, Paul. Healing with Whole Foods: Asian Traditions and Modern Nutrition. Berkeley, CA: North Atlantic Books, 2002; 465

25. Ibid., 356

HYDRATE

26. Sturm, Alison. "The Health Benefits of Dark Chocolate." Chocolate.com. 28 Oct. 2008 http://www.chocolate.com/articles/the-health-benefits-of-dark-chocolate.html

SNACK AND APPETIZE

27. Pitchford, Paul. Healing with Whole Foods: Asian Traditions and Modern Nutrition. Berkeley, CA: North Atlantic Books, 2002; 543

28. Ibid., 617

29. Ibid., 649

SIMMER WITH SOUP

30. Pitchford, Paul. Healing with Whole Foods: Asian Traditions and Modern Nutrition. Berkeley, CA: North Atlantic Books, 2002; 507

31. Ibid, 540, 544

32. Ibid., 507

33. Ibid., 296

34. Ibid., 549

35. Ibid., 228-229

36. Ibid., 509

37. Ibid., 539

SLOWLY WITH SALAD

38. Pitchford, Paul. Healing with Whole Foods: Asian Traditions and Modern Nutrition. Berkeley, CA: North Atlantic Books, 2002; 537

39. Ibid., 507

40. Ibid., 465

41. Ibid., 550

42. Ibid., 580

43. Ibid., 228-229

44. Ibid., 623

45. Ibid., 544

46. Ibid., 156

47. Ibid., 549

48. Ibid., 617

49. Ibid., 470

50. Ibid., 548

ON THE SIDE

51. Pitchford, Paul. Healing with Whole Foods: Asian Traditions and Modern Nutrition. Berkeley, CA: North Atlantic Books, 2002; 35

52. Pitchford, Paul. "Healing with Whole Foods." PowerPoint presentation. Heartwood Institute, Garberville, CA. August 2006

53. Ibid.

54. Pitchford, Paul. Healing with Whole Foods: Asian Traditions and Modern Nutrition. Berkeley, CA: North Atlantic Books, 2002; 551

55. Pitchford, Paul. Healing with Whole Foods: Asian Traditions and Modern Nutrition. Berkeley, CA: North Atlantic Books, 2002; 535

56. Ibid., 537

57. Ibid., 155

58. Ibid., 533

59. Ibid., 509

60. Ibid., 543

61. Willett, Walter C., Patrick J. Skerrett, and Jorge E. Chavarro. The Fertility Diet. New York: The McGraw-Hill Companies, 2007; 73

62. Ibid., 535

63. Lewis, Randine A. The Infertility Cure : The Ancient Chinese Wellness Program for Getting Pregnant and Having Healthy Babies. Boston: Little Brown & Company, 2005; 83

64. Pitchford, Paul. Healing with Whole Foods: Asian Traditions and Modern Nutrition. Berkeley, CA: North Atlantic Books, 2002; 538

65. Ibid., 537

66. Ibid., 659

MAIN ATTRACTION

67. Pitchford, Paul. Healing with Whole Foods: Asian Traditions and Modern Nutrition. Berkeley, CA: North Atlantic Books, 2002; 157

68. Ibid., 156

69. Ibid., 163

70. Ibid., 506-507

71. Ibid., 522

72. Ibid.,157

73. Ibid., 507

74. Ibid., 534

75. Ibid., 649

76. Ibid., 156

77. Ibid., 163

78. Ibid., 223

79. Ibid.,156

80. Ibid., 219

81. Ibid., 532

82. Ibid.,155

83. Ibid., 543

84. Ibid., 507

85. Ibid., 337

86. Ibid., 534

87. Ibid., 549

INDULGE

88. Pitchford, Paul. Healing with Whole Foods: Asian Traditions and Modern Nutrition. Berkeley, CA: North Atlantic Books, 2002; 356

Recipe Index

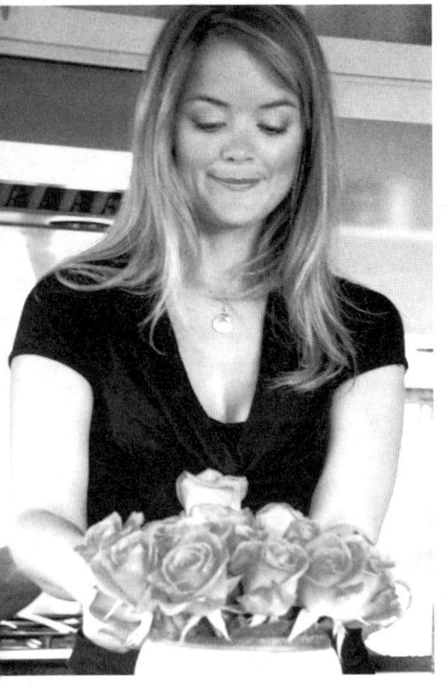

Acknowledgments

Sometimes we are graced by the presence of amazing teachers who change the way we look at the world. I have been blessed with two such people in the process of creating this book: Randine Lewis and Paul Pitchford. Randine Lewis generously shared her knowledge and love for the art of Chinese medicine as a mentor and a teacher on how people can enhance their fertility and the quality of their lives by reconnecting with their inherent nature. Paul Pitchford's commitment to educating on the power of healing with whole foods, along with tai chi, meditation and gentle living, is unparalleled. I have learned so much by studying with Randine and Paul and I am grateful to be able to share their wisdom with my clients and my family.

Many kind people contributed to making the recipes taste as good as they do. My amazing husband, Michael Flynn, graciously tested the recipes the whole way through and was especially patient in wading through some of the earliest renditions. I also want to thank my collaborator on the Cooking for Fertility DVD, Tiffany Pollard (Owner of EatingforEvolution.com), Caspar Poyck (Owner of ConsciouslyCulinary.com), Patty Papke and Patricia McKinell. Thank you to each of you for taking the time to infuse the recipes with your good energy.

I would also like to thank my family and the Fertile Soul staff and affiliates for their support in completing this project. Thank you to Cathy Doerken for introducing Randine and I. A special thank you to the editing team: Wendy Andersen, Laura Malone and Doug Yonson; to Gabriela Aparicio (info@gabrielamusic.com) for the cover and interior design; to Katy Saeger (SaegerMediaGroup.com) for being a wonderful part of the creative unfolding and to Kristen Bontadelli of Blinks Photography (blinksphotography@gmail.com) for the beautiful pictures in both the cookbook and the cooking DVD.

And finally, thanks to each of you who will share this book with clients, friends and family who are looking for greater health on their fertility journey.

With gratitude,

Kathryn

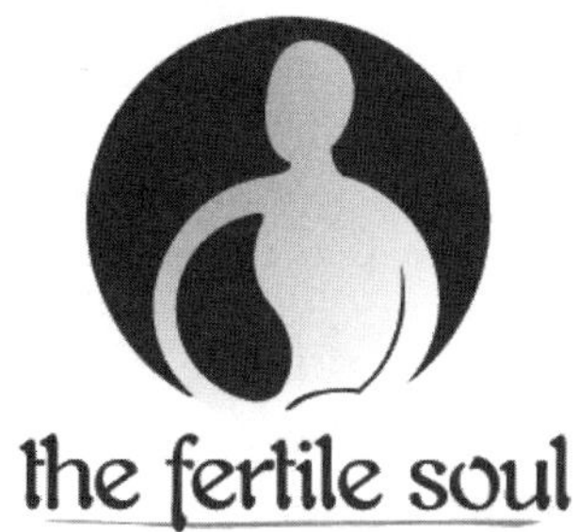

Fertile Soul Retreats

The Fertile Soul retreat process helps even the most challenging fertility cases achieve hope and healing. We are a Chinese-medicine based holistic program for body, mind, and spirit, to enhance your fertility and overcome obstructions to expressing your most fertile potential.

Dr. Randine Lewis personally takes individuals and couples into the depth of their healing potential, while teaching and reinforcing methods to heal the reproductive function. Dr. Lewis and her revolutionary retreat process has helped thousands of couples around the world conceive naturally and with the help of assisted reproductive technology. Most had given up hope before attending the retreat. Regardless of your fertility challenge, we are here to help.

Retreats are held monthly and space is limited. To find out more about The Fertile Soul retreat process, please visit us on our website, www.thefertilesoul.com.

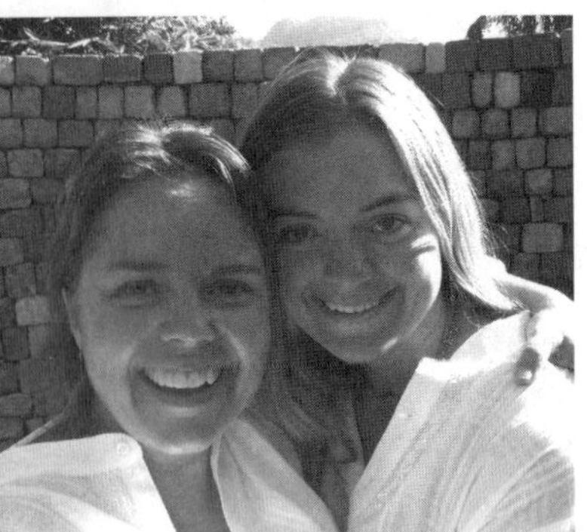

Randine and Kathryn at the Fertile Soul retreat at the Ananda Spa in India, 2005

About the Author

My journey through the wonderful world of holistic healing began when I had the opportunity to meet Randine Lewis, author of The Infertility Cure and The Way of the Fertile Soul. As a patient, I found that she confronted health issues that I had dealt with for years, and as a student I absorbed all of the wisdom she had to impart. And so my journey continued from Randine Lewis to studying with Paul Pitchford, author of Healing with Whole Foods. I have seen both sides, first as a patient and then as a practitioner. In both I found healing and truth in whole foods, relaxation, and many of the techniques of Chinese medicine. I believe that the bounty of the earth and wisdom of centuries passed can heal the damages wreaked on the female body by the stress and lifestyle of our modern world.

I experienced the healing power of a whole food diet and have been blessed to train and study with the foremost experts in the fields of women's health, whole food, and fertility. Today I use both Eastern and Western nutritional therapies in a multi-tiered approach that guides my clients toward improved levels of balanced health. For the past five years, I have led group lectures in nutrition education, five-element phase diagnosis, self-treatment through acupressure and fertility yoga. I provide individual nutritional counseling to men and women worldwide, with the intention of naturally enhancing reproductive capacity through a holistic approach that includes lifestyle changes, relaxation techniques, exercise and healing foods.

As founder of Fertile Foods.com my intention is to support women and men during the childbearing years by encouraging relaxation, pleasure, exercise, healthy foods and high-quality nutrient supplementation. I have also developed a line of MoonTime teas, to help women reconnect with the cyclical nature of the moon, our monthly cycles and nature. To learn more about Cooking for Fertility and to share recipes, please visit CookingforFertility.com.